Staying Fit

ISSUES

Volume 162

Series Editor

Lisa Firth

Independence

First published by Independence
The Studio, High Green
Great Shelford
Cambridge CB22 5EG
England

© Independence 2008

British Library Cataloguing in Publication Data
Staying Fit — (Issues Series)
I. Firth, Lisa II. Series
306.4'613

ISBN 978 1 86168 455 4

Printed in Great Britain
MWL Print Group Ltd

Cover
The illustration on the front cover is by
Don Hatcher.

CONTENTS

Chapter One: Unfit Britain

Chapter Two: Fitness Solutions

Useful information for readers

Dear Reader,

Issues: Staying Fit

Around one in four men and one in three women in the UK are overweight, and child obesity is also a major health issue. As well as risks for the individual which come with being overweight – including circulatory diseases, diabetes and some forms of cancer – obesity also affects society, with the cost of related health problems expected to cause a crisis in the NHS if trends continue. This book looks at how and why we should stay fit.

The purpose of *Issues*

Staying Fit is the one hundred and sixty-second volume in the **Issues** series. The aim of this series is to offer up-to-date information about important issues in our world. Whether you are a regular reader or new to the series, we do hope you find this book a useful overview of the many and complex issues involved in the topic. This title replaces an older volume in the **Issues** series, Volume 113: **Fitness and Health,** which is now out of print.

Titles in the **Issues** series are resource books designed to be of especial use to those undertaking project work or requiring an overview of facts, opinions and information on a particular subject, particularly as a prelude to undertaking their own research.

The information in this book is not from a single author, publication or organisation; the value of this unique series lies in the fact that it presents information from a wide variety of sources, including:
⇨ Government reports and statistics
⇨ Newspaper articles and features
⇨ Information from think-tanks and policy institutes
⇨ Magazine features and surveys
⇨ Website material
⇨ Literature from lobby groups and charitable organisations. *

Critical evaluation

Because the information reprinted here is from a number of different sources, readers should bear in mind the origin of the text and whether the source is likely to have a particular bias or agenda when presenting information (just as they would if undertaking their own research). It is hoped that, as you read about the many aspects of the issues explored in this book, you will critically evaluate the information presented. It is important that you decide whether you are being presented with facts or opinions. Does the writer give a biased or an unbiased report? If an opinion is being expressed, do you agree with the writer?

Staying Fit offers a useful starting point for those who need convenient access to information about the many issues involved. However, it is only a starting point. Following each article is a URL to the relevant organisation's website, which you may wish to visit for further information.

Kind regards,

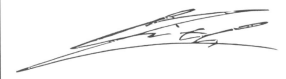

Lisa Firth
Editor, **Issues** series

* Please note that Independence Publishers has no political affiliations or opinions on the topics covered in the Issues series, and any views quoted in this book are not necessarily those of the publisher or its staff.

Obesity

Information from NetDoctor. Reviewed by Dr Roger Henderson, GP

What is obesity?

Obesity is more than just a few extra pounds.

Obesity is the heavy accumulation of fat in your body to such a degree that it rapidly increases your risk of diseases that can damage your health and knock years off your life, such as heart disease and diabetes.

The fat may be equally distributed around the body or concentrated on the stomach (apple-shaped) or the hips and thighs (pear-shaped).

For medical purposes, the body mass index (BMI) is used to determine if your weight is in the healthy range.

Work out your BMI

Take your weight (kg) and divide it by the square of your height (m).

For example, if you weigh 80kg and are 1.7m:

1 Multiply your height by itself 1.7x1.7=2.89
2 Divide your weight by this figure.
3 $80 \div 2.89 = 27.7 \text{kg/m}^2$.
4 27.7 is the BMI.

Doctors use BMI because it compares your weight against your height.

⇨ You are in the normal range if your BMI is between 18.5 and 25 (kg/m^2).
⇨ You are overweight if your BMI is between 25 and 30.
⇨ You are obese if your BMI is 30 or higher.
⇨ You are morbidly obese if your BMI is 40 or higher.

How common is obesity?

Around one in four men and one in three women in the UK are overweight, according to government statistics.

While slightly more women than men are obese (24 per cent versus 23 per cent), in the last ten years there has been a greater increase in the number of men who are obese.

The Department of Health predicts that if this trend continues, by 2010 around 6.6 million men will be obese compared to 6 million women.

Stomach obesity, where weight is concentrated on the tummy, is the most common type of obesity and affects 30 per cent of adult men.

Obesity and stomach obesity are rapidly increasing, especially in young people.

Around one in three children between the ages of 2 and 15 are overweight. While in total more girls than boys are overweight, a greater number of boys are obese.

⇨ 14 per cent of boys are overweight.
⇨ 17 per cent of girls are overweight.
⇨ 19 per cent of boys are obese.
⇨ 18 per cent of girls are obese.

Children and BMI

The BMI figures used in this article apply to adults only.

Doctors use special charts to work out BMI for children to take account of differing rates of growth and development.

Government statistics also show that children are more likely to have a weight problem if one parent is overweight, and this risk is increased if both parents are overweight or obese.

What problems can obesity cause?

Psychologically, being overweight can affect your body image and damage self-esteem. In some cases this can cause social anxiety and depression.

Common physical problems include:
⇨ difficulties breathing;
⇨ difficulties walking or running;
⇨ increased sweating;
⇨ pain in the knees and back;
⇨ skin conditions such as acne;
⇨ gallstones.

The following medical conditions are also more common in obese people than in those of normal weight:
⇨ high blood pressure;
⇨ high cholesterol;
⇨ diseases related to hardening of the arteries such as heart attack and stroke (cardiovascular disease).
⇨ type 2 diabetes;
⇨ some types of cancer.

These conditions are often known as obesity-related diseases and are

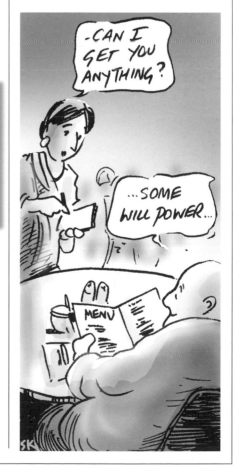

some of the most common causes of death before the age of 75. This is why obesity increases your risk of mortality.

What causes obesity?

Obesity can be hereditary, so some people are at increased risk.

Genetic factors can affect appetite, the rate at which you burn energy (metabolic rate) and how the body stores fat. Examples of genetic diseases are polycystic ovary syndrome (PCOS) and hypothyroidism.

But even if your genes make weight gain more likely, it is not inevitable that you will be overweight.

Obesity develops from:
⇨ overeating;
⇨ irregular meals;
⇨ lack of daily physical activity.

This is why obesity has trebled since 1980, when only 6 per cent of men and 8 per cent of women were obese. In this time our lifestyles have changed rapidly, with the ready availability of convenience foods and car journeys replacing walks to work and school.

It is lifestyle that determines how the genes develop.

Medicines such as antidepressants, corticosteroids and oral contraceptives can also cause weight gain.

When is obesity dangerous?

If you have a BMI of more than 25, you should lose weight. The same is true if you carry too much fat around the middle because this increases your risk of heart disease and diabetes.

UK clothes size

For women, the waistline target of 80cm means you should comfortably fit into a size 16.

Dress size	14	16	18	20
Waist (cm)	79	84	89	95
Dress size	22	24	26	
Waist (cm)	101	107	113	

Your waist should be no more than 102cm/40in (men) or 88cm/35in (women), with stricter targets for Asians of less than 90cm/35in (men) and 80cm/32in (women).

To reduce your risk of cardiovascular disease further, you should watch your waistline and make sure it's no more than 94cm/37in (men) and 80cm/32in (women).

How is obesity treated?

Initially, your doctor will suggest you lose weight through a change in diet and an increase in physical exercise.

Clinical guidelines are to aim for a weight loss of between 5kg and 10kg (11-22lb) over three months. This equals about 0.5kg or 1lb per week.

If you are obese, losing this amount will have a positive effect on your risk of cardiovascular disease and diabetes by reducing blood pressure, blood sugar (glucose) and cholesterol levels.

A dietitian can help you lose weight by giving nutritional advice on buying and preparing foods and designing a weight-loss plan.

Weight-loss plans are usually based on a low-fat diet of between 1500 and 2000 calories a day, which will result in a weight loss of 5 to 10kg in more than 90 per cent of obese people.

How do diet and exercise help?

Your body needs a certain amount of energy (calories) each day. Excess energy is stored as fat. The more active you are, the more calories your body needs.

By eating less than your body needs and exercising more, you force your body to use its existing fat stores for energy. By burning excess fat, you lose weight.

When is medical treatment necessary?

Your doctor will usually only consider medicines for weight loss if changes to diet and exercise are not effective.

Two medicines for weight-loss are available on the NHS: orlistat (Xenical) and sibutramine (Reductil).

Another weight-loss drug called rimonabant (Acomplia) has been recently launched, but until its cost-effectiveness has been assessed it is unlikely to be widely available on the NHS.

You will still need to follow a calorie-controlled diet and start an exercise plan while taking these drugs.

Treatment with Xenical and Reductil will only be continued after three months if you have lost 5 per cent of your body weight in that time.

While these medicines can help you to lose weight, there may be a gradual reversal of any weight loss after you stop treatment. To help avoid this, you will need to continue with changes to your diet and exercise levels.

Medicines for obesity are not yet recommended for young people under the age of 18 because we have no knowledge of possible negative

Definitions of overweight and obesity

The Body Mass Index (BMI) is the common method of evaluating individual people to see if they are under or overweight. It involves comparing their weight to their height by dividing the weight measurement (expressed in kilograms) by the square of the height (expressed in metres).

Classification	BMI (kg/m²): principal cut-off points
Underweight	**less than 18.50**
Severe thinness	less than 16.00
Moderate thinness	16.00-16.99
Mild thinness	17.00-18.49
Normal range	**18.50-24.99**
Overweight	**greater than or equal to 25.00**
Pre-obese	25.00-29.99
Obese	**greater than or equal to 30.00**
Obese class I	30.00-34.99
Obese class II	35.00 -39.99
Obese class III	greater than or equal to 40.00

Source: adapted from WHO, 1995, WHO, 2000 and WHO, 2004.

effects on puberty and later eating behaviour.

Orlistat (Xenical)
Xenical reduces the amount of fat that is absorbed from the bowels.

Your doctor can prescribe this drug if you are obese, or if your BMI is higher than 28 and you have a related risk factor such as high blood pressure, high cholesterol or diabetes.

Common side-effects include headache, urgent or increased need to open the bowels, flatulence (wind) with discharge, and oily or fatty stools.

Sibutramine (Reductil)
Reductil acts on chemicals in the brain called serotonin and noradrenaline to make you feel fuller for longer.

Your doctor can prescribe this drug if you are obese or have a BMI higher than 27 with a risk factor for heart disease, and you haven't been able to lose weight through lifestyle change within the last three months.

Common side-effects include loss of appetite, constipation, dry mouth and problems sleeping.

Rimonabant (Acomplia)
Acomplia is a new drug that blocks CB1 receptors in the brain and fat tissues that control appetite and the desire for sweet and fatty foods. This reduces appetite and cravings for these types of foods.

A doctor can prescribe this drug if you are obese or have a BMI higher than 27 with a risk factor for heart disease.

Common side-effects include nausea and infections of the upper airways.

What about weight reduction surgery?
You can be considered for weight-loss surgery if you are morbidly obese, or if you have a BMI between 35 and 40 and have a risk factor for an obesity-related disease.

This type of surgery is known as bariatric surgery.

Gastric banding
Gastric banding or 'lap banding' limits the capacity of the stomach so you feel full after eating a small amount of food.

Keyhole surgery is used to tie an inflatable band around the top part of the stomach, creating a small pouch

at the top. This limits the amount of food your stomach can hold.

Food then slowly passes from the pouch into the lower part of your stomach and on into your digestive system.

The operation is reversible.

Gastric bypass
Gastric bypass is permanent surgery on the stomach to reduce the length of the digestive tract and stop food being absorbed.

> ## Obesity is the heavy accumulation of fat in your body to such a degree that it rapidly increases your risk of diseases that can damage your health and knock years off your life

---

A small pouch is created at the top of the stomach.

Part of the intestine is then grafted to the top of this pouch so food bypasses the stomach and much of the intestine, meaning it can't be digested.

Gastric balloon insertion
Gastric balloon insertion is a less permanent type of surgery. It is not widely available on the NHS.

A balloon is placed on the end of a thin, flexible tube called an endoscope. It is inserted into your stomach via your mouth.

Liquid or air is then pumped into the balloon so it partially fills the stomach. This creates a feeling of fullness.

The balloon is usually removed after six months.

Complications of weight-loss surgery include the usual risks of surgery and long-term digestive problems such as nausea, heartburn, vomiting and diarrhoea.

After surgery your body absorbs less food, but it will also absorb less vitamins and nutrients. This means you are at greater risk of diseases caused by vitamin and mineral deficiency such as anaemia and osteoporosis.

In the long term
While plenty of diets and slimming products claim to offer quick fixes, obesity is not something that can be cured or brought under clinical control within a few weeks or months.

Treatment such as diet and exercise may need to continue for years.

Weight-loss plans from a GP or dietitian are an effective way to lose weight, but a greater challenge is to achieve a way of life that maintains weight and reduces the chances of putting it back on.

This can only be achieved by permanently changing your eating and exercise habits.

Further information
⇨ BOSPA (British Obesity Surgery Patient Association) has information on many types of weight-loss surgery: www.bospa.org

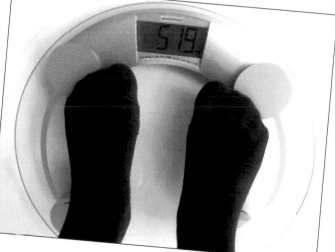

⇨ National Obesity Forum: www. nationalobesityforum.org.uk
Based on a text by Professor Arne Astrup
Last updated 30 August 2007

⇨ The above information is reprinted with kind permission from NetDoctor. Visit www.netdoctor. co.uk for more information.
© NetDoctor

The politics of obesity

Information from politics.co.uk

What is obesity?

A minority medical condition 50 years ago, the prevalence of obesity is now such that it is regarded as a major public health issue and listed as a priority by senior government ministers.

A person is considered obese when their body weight reaches an excessive level. In the UK, clinicians generally use the Body Mass Index (BMI) to measure obesity. BMI is obtained by dividing a person's weight in kilograms by their height in metres squared. A BMI between 18.5 and 25 is considered 'normal'. A BMI over 25 is classed as 'overweight' and a person is obese once their BMI reaches 30.

Obesity as a public health issue does not seek to make aesthetic judgements about people carrying extra body fat. Obesity is linked to a number of illnesses and reduced lifespan and the government is keen to reduce the prevalence of obesity among the population.

Background

Obesity is a relatively modern phenomenon; whereas past governments were concerned with inadequate nutrition and underweight children, politicians now launch initiatives against childhood obesity and encourage voters to slim down.

Now nearly a quarter of adults in England are obese, with obesity having tripled since the 1980s. By 2050 it is estimated that 60 per cent of men and 50 per cent of women will be severely overweight. Obesity among children has also increased to unprecedented levels.

Being overweight used to be seen as a personal medical complaint, largely blamed on genetics or constitution. The rising prevalence of obesity has forced health professionals and politicians to consider the lifestyle factors contributing to expanding waistlines.

It is now generally accepted that an imbalance between energy consumed in the form of calories and energy used causes weight gain or loss. This means sedentary lifestyles combined with the easy availability of calorie-rich foods presuppose a population towards obesity.

> **A minority medical condition 50 years ago, the prevalence of obesity is now such that it is regarded as a major public health issue and listed as a priority by senior government ministers**

Just a third of men and a quarter of women claim to achieve the recommended 30 minutes of exercise five times a week. Half of those not taking part claim their health is not good enough to exercise and nearly one in five say they do not have time. Working patterns have seen Britons shift to office-based jobs and longer working hours at the same time as rising obesity levels.

The prevalence of fast food chains and cheap, nutritionally poor food has led many to blame diet for rising obesity and many health campaigns focus on the importance of low-fat or low-calorie food choices. Although this is a commonsense approach it should be noted that total energy intake fell by 20 per cent between 1974 and 2004, precisely those years when obesity soared.

Politicians are concerned by obesity because of the effect it appears to have on a person's general health – and the resultant pressure of this on health services. Obesity has been linked to an increased risk of heart disease, type 2 diabetes and some cancers. Excessive weight is blamed for 9,000 premature deaths a year in England and is estimated to reduce life expectancy by an average of nine years. The government calculates that obesity costs the NHS £1 billion a year, with a further economic cost of £2.3 billion to £2.6 billion.

Controversy

The government has unapologetically defined obesity as a symptom of ill health which should be eradicated. Attempting to manipulate individuals' weight leaves the government vulnerable to accusations of 'nanny statism'.

The UK is yet to see the rise of a significant 'fat positive' movement. In the US a minority of obese people have

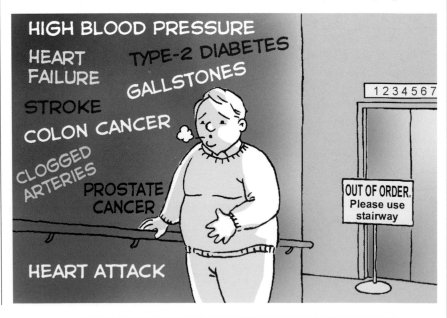

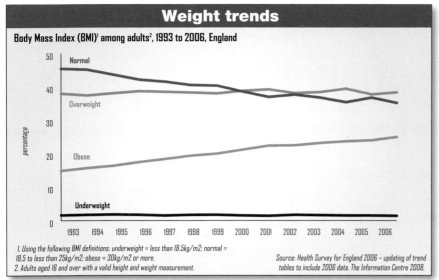

Weight trends

Body Mass Index (BMI)[1] among adults[2], 1993 to 2006, England

1. Using the following BMI definitions: underweight = less than 18.5kg/m2; normal = 18.5 to less than 25kg/m2; obese = 30kg/m2 or more.
2. Adults aged 16 and over with a valid height and weight measurement.

Source: Health Survey for England 2006 – updating of trend tables to include 2006 data. The Information Centre 2008.

hit out at attempts to medicalise and stigmatise their size and argue societies should accept people of all weights.

While most people accept that extreme fatness is not desirable, many are more resistant towards government attempts to enforce healthy lifestyles. At the extreme end this has seen parents feed burgers to their children through school gates after the government enforced new healthier school meals.

The public may resent government attempts to encourage healthy eating but the government has in turn been criticised for failing to promote or enable healthy lifestyles. Many point out it is inconsistent for ministers to lecture school children about healthy lunch choices while allowing the sale of school playing fields. Infrastructure such as cycle lanes is also poor in the UK compared to other European nations and many claim that private gyms remain prohibitively expensive.

A correlation can be observed between socio-economic status and obesity, although at least one recent study has found this is less pronounced among children. This has led many to interpret obesity as a symptom of health inequality. Although many commentators do note factors such as the price of gym membership, much of the blame for higher levels of obesity among poor people is placed on dietary choices.

Politicians and chefs are just some of those debating whether it really is cheaper to eat badly. In a bid to counter the assumption that junk food is more cost effective, ministers have been asked to consider the option of 'fat taxes' whereby a charge is levied against high fat, high salt or high sugar foods. This suggestion has proved incredibly unpopular with the public.

Despite the acceptance that too many calories and not enough activity will cause weight gain, scientists are still searching for a 'fat gene'. The diet industry has proved highly inefficient in the long term, with most dieters either struggling to lose weight or putting it back on when lost. Nevertheless the government is determined the rising prevalence of obesity can be reversed.

How obesity is measured has also been criticised, with the BMI dismissed by some as an imperfect science. The BMI fails to distinguish between body fat and lean muscle, meaning professional athletes can emerge as overweight or even obese. Moreover, it fails to look at where fat is distributed on the body. It is now recognised that excess fat around the abdomen is a greater health risk than fat on the buttocks or thighs. For this reason, the World Health Organisation now recommends people measure their waists. A circumference over 37 inches (94 cm) on a man or 32 inches (80 cm) on a woman indicates a health risk.

Some have also questioned the assumption that excessive weight is a health risk. Obesity does broadly correlate to increased rates of a range of illnesses including diabetes and a number of cancers. However, a review of 7,000 studies by the World Cancer Research Fund found a third of cancers are attributable to diet and found at least six cancers for which obesity was a major risk factor.

However, it has been pointed out that these could also be caused by the lifestyle typically enjoyed by obese people, rather than the excess fat per se. It is, some argue, possible to be overweight and healthy. A recent study in the *Journal of American Medical Association* contradicted received wisdom by concluding extra weight could prolong life span.

Statistics

⇨ In 2005, 22 per cent of men and 24 per cent of women were obese.
⇨ By 2050 this is expected to increase to 60 per cent of men and 50 per cent of women.
⇨ 18 per cent of boys and girls aged 2 to 15 years old are obese in England. In 1995, this was 11 per cent and 12 per cent respectively.
⇨ If one million people lost weight, 15,000 fewer people a year would develop coronary heart disease, 34,000 fewer people type 2 diabetes and 99,000 fewer people would develop high blood pressure.
⇨ 26 per cent of men and 30 per cent of women eat at least five servings of fruit and vegetables a day. This has increased since 2001.

Statistics 1-3 & 5: (Source: Department of Health, 2007); statistic 4: (Source: National Audit Office, 2007).

Quotes

'Obesity is associated with many illnesses and is directly related to increased mortality and lower life expectancy. Tackling obesity is a government wide priority.'
Department of Health, 2007.

'We are facing a potential crisis on the scale of climate change and it is in everybody's interest to turn things round. There is no single solution to tackle obesity and it cannot be tackled by government action alone.'
Alan Johnson, secretary of state for health, 2007.
14 November 2007

⇨ The above information is reprinted with kind permission from politics.co.uk. Visit www.politics.co.uk for more information.
© *politics.co.uk*

Statistics on obesity, physical activity and diet

Main findings

Obesity

⇨ In 2006, 24% of adults (aged 16 or over) in England were classified as obese. This represents an overall increase from 15% in 1993.

⇨ Men and women were equally likely to be obese, however women were more likely than men to be morbidly obese (3% compared to 1%).

⇨ Thirty-seven per cent of adults had a raised waist circumference in 2006 compared to 23% in 1993. Women were more likely then men to have a raised waist circumference (41% and 32% respectively).

⇨ Using both BMI and waist circumference to assess risk of health problems, of men 20% were estimated to be at increased risk, 13% at high risk and 21% at very high risk. Equivalent figures for women were 14% at increased risk, 16% at high risk and 23% at very high risk.

⇨ In 2006, 16% of children aged 2 to 15 were classed as obese. This represents an overall increase from 11% in 1995. Despite the overall increase since 1995, the proportion of girls aged 2 to 15 who were obese decreased between 2005 and 2006, from 18% to 15%. There was no significant decrease among boys aged 2 to 15 over that period. Among children aged 2 to 10, 15% were classed as obese in 2006.

⇨ Boys were more likely than girls to be obese (17% compared to 15%).

⇨ Of children aged 8 to 15 who were classed as obese, two-thirds (66%) of girls and 60% of boys thought that they were too heavy.

Physical activity

⇨ Overall, physical activity has increased among both men and women since 1997, with 40% of men and 28% of women meeting the recommended levels in 2006 (at least 30 minutes of at least moderate intensity activity at least 5 times a week).

⇨ There is a clear gradient across the income quintiles for both men and women, with those in the lowest income quintile more likely to be in the low participation group than those in the highest income quintile. Those with the highest income were also most likely to participate in active sport: 89% of those earning over £50k had done so at least once in the previous 12 months while for those whose income was less than £10k the figure was 61%.

⇨ Men and women with low physical activity levels were more than twice as likely as to have a raised waist circumference than those with high levels of physical activity.

⇨ Three in ten adults had not participated in active sport in the last 12 months in 2005/06. The main reasons for not participating were 'health isn't good enough' (47%) followed by 'difficulty in finding the time' and 'not being interested' (both 18%).

⇨ In 2006, boys were more likely than girls to meet the recommended levels of physical activity with 70% of boys and 59% of girls reporting taking part in 60 minutes or more of physical activity on all 7 days in the previous week.

⇨ During 2006/07, 86% of pupils took part in at least two hours of high quality PE and sport a week, a gradual increase since 2003/04 when the figure was 62%.

Diet

⇨ In 2006, 28% of men and 32% of women consumed five or more portions of fruit and vegetables a day, the proportion doing so generally increases with age and income.

⇨ Among children aged 5 to 15, in 2006, 19% of boys and 22% of girls consumed five or more portions of fruit and vegetables a day.

⇨ The proportion of adults and children consuming five or more portions of fruit and vegetables a day remained steady between 2001 and 2004. There were increases among adults in 2005 and 2006. For children, there was an increase among both boys and girls in 2005 and further increase among girls in 2006.

Health outcomes

⇨ For people aged 35 and over classified as having a raised waist circumference, men were twice as likely and women were four times more likely to have type 2 diabetes.

⇨ Over the last ten years there were 17,458 Finished Consultant Episodes (FCEs) with a primary diagnosis of obesity. Almost a quarter of these (4,068) occurred in 2006/07.

⇨ In 2006, 1.06 million prescription items were dispensed for the treatment of obesity. Overall, the number of prescriptions in 2006 was more than eight times the number prescribed in 1999, when there were 127 thousand prescription items. Considering the treatment types in 2006, around 73% of prescriptions were for Orlistat and 25% prescriptions were for Sibutramine, the two main drugs used for treatment of obesity.

January 2008

⇨ The above information is reprinted with kind permission from the NHS. Visit www.ic.nhs.uk for more information.

Obesity worldwide

Information from the World Heart Federation

Obesity across the world

⇨ Worldwide, 400 million adults are obese and 1.6 billion are overweight.

⇨ Worldwide, 155 million children are overweight, including 30-45 million obese children.

⇨ Obesity levels have risen sharply across the globe. Even in those countries that have historically had lower rates of obesity, there is now evidence of increasing overweight.

⇨ In the Americas, the United States is by far the fattest country: 31% of adult males and 33% of adult females are obese.

⇨ Croatia has the largest portion of obese men in Europe, at 31%, and Albania the most obese women, 36%.

⇨ In Lebanon, 36% of men are obese, the highest proportion in the Eastern Mediterranean and Jordan has the highest female incidence at 60%.

⇨ The most obese nations of the world are in the Western Pacific:
  ↳ in Nauru 80% of men are obese, 78% of women;
  ↳ in Tonga 47% of men and 70% of women are obese;
  ↳ in Samoa 33% of men are obese and 63% of women.

Why obesity rates have risen

⇨ People have become fatter because increased calorie intake is not offset by increased physical inactivity; in fact, globally humanity is becoming more physically inactive.

⇨ Diets have moved from being plant-based to high-fat, energy-dense animal-based diets.

Obesity and cardiovascular disease

⇨ Being overweight raises the risk of developing high blood pressure, diabetes and stiff, clogged arteries, all risk factors for cardiovascular diseases (CVD).

⇨ As an individual's overweight increases so does the risk of developing CVD.

How obesity causes CVD

⇨ Fat, stored in the torso, affects blood pressure, the fat levels in the blood, and interferes with the body's ability to use insulin effectively.

⇨ Failure to properly use insulin can lead to the development of type 2 diabetes, a risk factor of CVD.

Changes in eating habits

⇨ Since the 60s the average daily calorie intake has increased across the globe.

⇨ The consumption of foods high in fats and sweeteners is increasing throughout the developing world, while the share of cereals is declining; intake of fruits and vegetables remains inadequate.

⇨ Families in industrialised nations spend more of their money than ever before on meals purchased away from home.

⇨ Commercially prepared food is higher in fat and sugar.

⇨ The portions in fast food restaurants across the globe are between 2 to 5 times larger than 2 decades ago.

⇨ In the US snacking contributes about one-fifth of total daily energy for adolescents and is excess calories.

⇨ In the US consumption of chips/crackers/popcorn/pretzels tripled from the mid-1970s to the mid-1990s and soft drinks intake doubled.

⇨ In 2006, 150,000 new foods and drinks products were launched worldwide; that is 300 new products appeared in stores around the globe each day.

May 2007

⇨ The above information is reprinted with kind permission from the World Heart Federation. Visit www.world-heart-federation.org to view references for this article or for more information on the relationship between fitness and a healthy heart.

© *World Heart Federation*

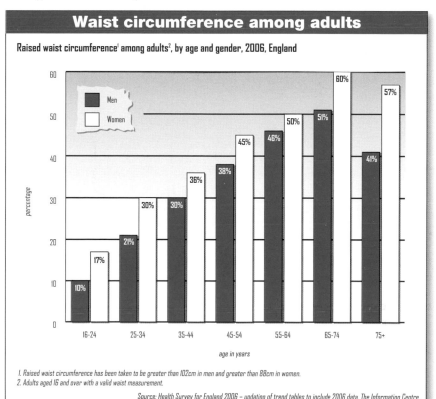

Waist circumference among adults

Raised waist circumference[1] among adults[2], by age and gender, 2006, England

1. Raised waist circumference has been taken to be greater than 102cm in men and greater than 88cm in women.
2. Adults aged 16 and over with a valid waist measurement.

Source: Health Survey for England 2006 – updating of trend tables to include 2006 data. The Information Centre.

Fat attack

Why we get fat

Whereas older generations can still remember the reality of ration books during and after the Second World War, younger Britons have grown up accustomed to food in plenty, at all times. But even at the height of rationing, when desirable foods such as meat, chocolate and sugar were in short supply, people rarely went hungry. We in the West are fortunate enough to see famine and starvation as the problems of a bygone era, or another continent.

Between the car, the office, the sofa, the supermarket and the microwave, we do not expend as much energy as we once did

---

But our bodies have longer memories.

The legacy of evolution

In our evolutionary history consistent food supplies were far from certain. To eat you had to hunt or gather edible vegetation. With the supply of such meals inevitably being subject to the vagaries of nature and luck, our ancestors lived with the real possibility of starvation. So it is not surprising that our bodies learned to stockpile food when it was abundant, in anticipation of harder times.

This evolutionary legacy remains with us today. Food provides the energy the body needs to carry out the metabolic processes that keep us alive, including the very process of digesting food, as well as breathing and the heartbeat. It also provides the fuel for anything else that we do, such as walking and talking. We measure this energy in units called calories and kilocalories (1,000 calories). Confusingly, when we refer to calories in everyday conversation, what we actually mean is kilocalories.

When we eat more food than we need, the body stores any extra calories, just in case. These are normally stored as fat, because, weight for weight, fat can store almost twice the calories that carbohydrates and proteins can. One kilogram of fat stores approximately 9,000 kilocalories.

What is fat?

Fat is an umbrella term for a number of chemical compounds that are stable, not soluble in water, and oily or greasy to the touch. Together with oils, they comprise one of the three principal classes of foodstuffs, the others being proteins and carbohydrates. Nearly all plant and animal cells contain these basic substances, though in different quantities. Nut kernels can be up to 70% fat, while a white potato is less than 0.1% fat.

In the body, special cells called adipose cells store large globules of fat. Together, these cells form adipose tissue – large reservoirs of fat cells – mainly beneath the skin, but also around the organs of the body.

Apart from being the principal medium for storing energy in the body, fat has other valuable functions. The fatty adipose tissue around our organs acts as cushioning protection, while the fat under our skin insulates us from the cold. Fat is also vital for storing and transporting important fat-soluble vitamins (A, D, E and K) in the body, and for maintaining healthy skin and hair.

Calorie counting

Between the car, the office, the sofa, the supermarket and the microwave, we do not expend as much energy as we once did. And we eat far more regularly. Though necessary energy intake changes with age and lifestyle, it is recommended that women eat between 2,000 and 2,500 kilocalories a day, and men between 2,500 and 3,000 kilocalories a day. If we eat more than this, or use less than this, the extra is stored away as fat. And if we regularly store fat away, and rarely plunder our reserves, we end up being overweight.

No excuses

Why some people are fatter than others is less of a mystery than many of us would like to believe. That some people put on fat more readily than others is true. But this is more likely to be related to a greater interest in food, or a less energetic lifestyle, than to genetics, hormones, or metabolic rates.

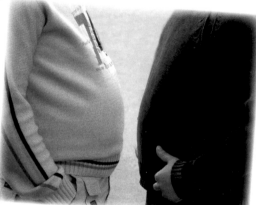

Obesity can run in families, but even this may be the result of early feeding patterns taught by parent to child rather than a genetic predisposition to fat accumulation. Such patterns can apply to nations as well as families. Affluent populations like our own and that of the US have an abundant supply of high-calorie foods, and increasingly sedentary living habits, which can easily lead to patterns of over-eating and consequent obesity.

Of all the factors that contribute to obesity, hormonal and glandular defects are thought to be the least important, being demonstrable in only about 5% of all obese individuals.

⇨ The above information is reprinted with kind permission from Channel 4. Visit www.channel4.com for more information.

© Channel 4

Genetic risk of obesity

Gene sequence puts half of UK population at greater risk of obesity, researchers say

⇨ *Discovery could suggest ways to curb epidemic.*
⇨ *Problem most common in Indian-origin Britons.*

By Ian Sample, Science Correspondent

A section of genetic code that puts half the population at greater risk of obesity, diabetes and heart disease has been discovered by scientists who say those carrying the sequence are on average 2kg (4.4lb) heavier than others, with 2cm larger waistlines and a tendency to become resistant to insulin and vulnerable to late-onset diabetes.

While 50% of the UK population carries the obesity-related sequence, it is a third more common among people of Indian Asian ancestry than among Europeans, the scientists said.

The finding raises hopes of new measures to curb the soaring obesity rates, including genetic screening programmes to identify children most at risk of what has become one of the leading causes of poor health and mortality in the developed world.

'A better understanding of the genes behind problems such as diabetes and cardiovascular disease means that we will be in a good position to identify people whose genetic inheritance makes them most susceptible,' said Professor Jaspal Kooner, lead author of the study at Imperial College London. 'We can't change their genetic inheritance, but we can focus on preventative

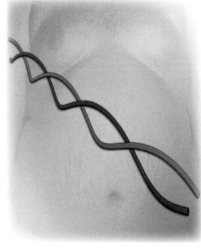

Are genetics responsible for obesity?

measures, including lifestyle factors such as diet and exercise.'

By unravelling the genetics of obesity, scientists believe that ultimately they will be able to develop therapies for the condition.

Obesity rates in Britain have almost quadrupled in the past 25 years, making the country the most obese in Europe. More than one in five men and a quarter of women in Britain are now clinically obese. Each year, an estimated 30,000 people in England alone die prematurely from obesity-related conditions such as diabetes, heart disease and cancer.

The research was carried out as part of the London Life Sciences Population project into the environmental and genetic causes of obesity, diabetes and heart disease. To find the gene sequence, scientists analysed the genetic make-up of 30,000 British citizens of European and Indian Asian ancestry and looked for markers that were common only among those with obesity.

The section of genetic code lies close to a gene called MC4R, which is know to control energy levels in the body by regulating how much food we eat and how much energy we burn. The team believe the gene sequence controls the activity of the MC4R gene, which has previously been linked to rare and extreme cases of childhood obesity.

'Until now, we have understood remarkably little about the genetic component of common problems linked with obesity, such as cardiovascular disease and diabetes. Finding such a close association between a genetic sequence and significant physical effects is very important, especially when the sequence is found

in half the population,' Kooner said.

The discovery that the gene sequence is more common among people of Indian Asian ancestry could explain the unusually high rates of obesity and insulin resistance in this group, which makes up 25% of the world's population but is expected to account for 40% of global heart disease by 2020.

Last year, scientists reported that people who inherited a particular form of a gene called FTO were 70% more likely to be obese than those who did not. Like MC4R, the FTO gene is thought to influence appetite and how much energy the body uses.

Taken together, the FTO variant and MC4R gene sequence increase body weight by 4-5kg.

In a second paper, researchers from Oxford University and the Wellcome Trust's Sanger Institute in Cambridge also link a gene sequence close to MC4R with obesity. Their study, based on 90,000 people in Sweden, found that those inheriting the section of DNA were 1.5kg heavier than others.

The study, led by Inës Barroso, at the Sanger Institute, found a dramatic difference between the effect the obesity genes had in childhood and adulthood. Between the ages of four and seven, children gained almost twice as much weight as adults, almost entirely by developing more fat, the scientists found.

'The precise role in obesity of genetic variants in FTO and near MC4R remains to be discovered, but we can now begin to understand the biological consequences of these,' Barroso said.

Government strategy

Alan Johnson, the health secretary, described obesity as 'the most significant public and personal health problem facing our society' when he unveiled the government's five-point plan for tackling the country's weight problem earlier this year.

The government's strategy aims to encourage healthier lifestyles by raising awareness of nutrition, such as the advice to eat five portions of fruit and vegetables a day, and by promoting daily physical activity.

Under the plans, junk food has been banned from school vending machines, and cookery classes are due to be made compulsory in a majority of schools in September. The government is also considering clamping down on the construction of fast-food outlets close to schools and parks.

Another strand of the strategy aims to help people cut their intake of saturated fats, salt and sugar, a move that could see the food industry come under pressure to adopt single food labelling systems. The plans include talks with the entertainment industry to find ways for parents to limit how much time children spend watching TV and playing computer games.

5 May 2008

© *Guardian Newspapers Limited 2008*

Sleepwalking towards obesity

Modern life has the UK sleepwalking towards obesity

The technological revolution of the 20th century has led to weight gain becoming inevitable for most people, because our bodies and biological make-up are out of step with our surroundings, says the latest report from Foresight, the government's futures think tank.

The technological revolution of the 20th century has led to weight gain becoming inevitable

The study found that obesity has many causes and is a much more passive phenomenon than is often assumed. Our basic biological instincts combined with our modern environment means that we're destined to put on weight. The research found that the problem of obesity will take at least 30 years to reverse.

The 'Tackling Obesities: Future Choices' Foresight project, sponsored by the Public Health Minister, Dawn Primarolo, was an in-depth two-year study by almost 250 experts and scientists to examine the causes of obesity and map future trends to help government plan effective policies both now and in the future.

Foresight's diverse evidence shows that only a comprehensive long-term strategy will have an impact on the rising trends of obesity. Alignment with other policy goals such as climate change,

social inclusion and wellbeing is vital. Preventing obesity requires major change – in the environment and in behaviour; in organisations as well as in communities, families and individuals.

Sir David King, the government's Chief Scientific Adviser and head of the Foresight Programme, believes a wholesale change in attitudes towards obesity is required.

'Foresight has for the first time drawn together complex evidence to show that we must fight the notion that the current obesity epidemic arises from individual over-indulgence or laziness alone. Personal responsibility is important, but our study shows the problem is much more complicated. It is a wake-up call for the nation, showing that only change across many elements of our society will help us tackle obesity.

'Stocking up on food was key to survival in prehistoric times, but now with energy dense, cheap foods, labour-saving devices, motorised transport and sedentary work, obesity is rapidly becoming a consequence of modern life.'

As part of the CSR announcement the government signalled a new long-term ambition to tackle obesity across the population as part of the new Child health PSA to improve the health and wellbeing of children and young people.

Tackling childhood obesity remains a key cross-government priority as part of this wider ambition: Our ambition is to reverse the rising tide of obesity and overweight in the population, by enabling everyone to achieve and

Key findings

⇨ Most adults in the UK are already overweight. Modern living ensures every generation is heavier than the last – 'Passive Obesity'.

⇨ By 2050 60% of men and 40% of women could be clinically obese. Without action, obesity-related diseases will cost an extra £45.5 billion per year.

⇨ The obesity epidemic cannot be prevented by individual action alone and demands a societal approach.

⇨ Tackling obesity requires far greater change than anything tried so far, and at multiple levels: personal, family, community and national.

⇨ Preventing obesity is a societal challenge, similar to climate change. It requires partnership between government, science, business and civil society.

maintain a healthy weight. Our initial focus will be on children: By 2020, we aim to reduce the proportion of overweight and obese children to 2000 levels.

17 October 2007

⇨ The above information is reprinted with kind permission from Directgov. Visit www.direct.gov.uk for more information.

© *Crown copyright*

Busy lifestyles cause a death every 15 minutes

Information from the British Heart Foundation

Every 15 minutes someone dies as a direct result of physical inactivity. Yet just 30 minutes of activity a day will help stave off heart disease and other illnesses, the British Heart Foundation says today as it launches a new poster campaign.

Almost a third of people asked give lack of time as a reason for their inactivity, a new YouGov poll reveals. But three out of four would choose a sedentary activity such as using their computer, watching TV or reading if they had a spare 30 minutes in the day.

The survey results are published today as the BHF launches its celebrity-backed 30 a Day campaign featuring light-hearted billboard adverts showing combinations of everyday ways to be active such as washing the car, gardening or swimming.

With a growing ageing population in the UK, the campaign urges people who are 50 or over to get active now, in any way that suits them, to keep healthy and independent in their later life.

Dr Mike Knapton, Director of Prevention and Care at the BHF, says: 'It's an alarming thought that inactivity kills someone in the UK every 15 minutes. These deaths are avoidable and the solution is simple and achievable.

People who take regular physical activity have twice the protection against coronary heart disease as those who are inactive

---

'We can all make excuses, but at the end of the day it's up to individuals to make the change, to get up and to get active. Just 30 minutes a day can make all the difference, and it can be fun!

'Keeping fit doesn't have to mean sweating it out at the gym and it's never too late to start.'

As part of the campaign, the BHF is sending 2.5 million leaflets to households across the UK and the campaign poster will go up on over 2000 billboards across the UK.

People are urged to visit the campaign website, bhf.org.uk/30aday for practical, fun ways to be physically active, or to order a free campaign booklet by calling 0808 156 5630.

Top tips
⇨ The BHF recommends adults take 30 minutes of moderate physical activity on at least five days of the week.
⇨ The 30 minutes can be broken into 10- or 15-minute sessions.
⇨ As long as the activity makes you feel warm and breathe harder it will benefit your health.
⇨ All sorts of everyday activities can count towards your 30 a Day:
　↳ Walking is the easiest way to keep fit, and it's free! Just try upping your speed to a brisk walk.
　↳ Vacuum cleaning the house keeps your heart healthy, your carpets clean and earns you brownie points at home.
　↳ Tossing a Frisbee this summer is a fun, sociable and cheap way to get your 30 a Day.

The facts
⇨ People who take regular physical activity have twice the protection against coronary heart disease as those who are inactive.
⇨ Just 30% of UK 50- to 64-year-olds take the recommended amount of physical activity. And it gets worse as people get older – only 6% of 65- to 84-year-olds in England get enough exercise.
⇨ Three out of five 50- to 65-year-olds know what the recommended amount of exercise is, but they still choose to shun the health advice.

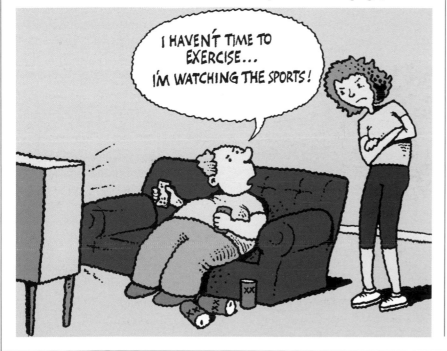

- ⇨ Over half this age group are worried they are not getting enough physical activity.
- ⇨ With regular, frequent exercise, people can dramatically improve their heart health as well as their mobility, balance and mental well-being, setting them up for a long and fulfilling later life.

The celebrities

Health-conscious celebrities who are backing the campaign include world darts champion, Phil 'The Power' Taylor, broadcaster Angela Rippon, comedian and world traveller Michael Palin, actress Lesley Joseph, actor Brian Blessed, TV personality Gloria Hunniford, Olympian Tessa Sanderson and actor Christopher Timothy.

- ⇨ Phil 'The Power' Taylor says: 'I was determined to get fitter – not only to improve my stamina in darts but also so I could enjoy being with my family, especially my grandson. I feel 100 times better since I started to exercise and know I will keep it up because it has given me a new lease of life.'
- ⇨ Michael Palin reveals how he keeps fit: 'For the past 25 years I've tried to run regularly, say three times a week. I only run against myself, so I don't have to be too competitive. It keeps me in shape and clears my mind as well.'
- ⇨ Angela Rippon gives her tips: 'Finding your own way to enjoy being physically active is key – be it dancing, swimming, long country walks – or whatever suits you. It's an investment in your future health, which you will never ever regret!'

The politics

Promoting good health among older adults must be a national priority. The BHF, working with the National Coalition on Active Ageing, are urging the government, health professionals, employers and the fitness industry to work together to help over-50s get active.

MPs will be presented with a policy 'blueprint' outlining the challenges and recommended targets at the Houses of Parliament on Wednesday (25 April).

The BHF calls on:
- ⇨ Government to run campaigns to get over-50s active.
- ⇨ Doctors to routinely refer patients to physical activity programmes.
- ⇨ Local authorities to build safe and 'walkable' towns.
- ⇨ Businesses to invest in activity schemes for older staff.
- ⇨ Fitness industry and sports clubs to run sessions for over-50s.

23 April 2007

⇨ The above information is re-printed with kind permission from the British Heart Foundation. Visit www.bhf.org.uk for more information.

© British Heart Foundation

Fitness and ageing

Sedentary lifestyle linked to faster ageing

People who do plenty of exercise appear to be biologically younger than those who lead a sedentary lifestyle, researchers have found.

Lack of exercise is already known to increase a person's risk of heart disease, high blood pressure, obesity, type-2 diabetes and some forms of cancer.

Now, researchers at King's College London have found visible signs of cellular ageing in people who are inactive.

The team studied 2,401 twins who were asked to provide a DNA sample and details of their activity levels, smoking habits and socioeconomic status.

The researchers then examined the length of telomeres – sections of DNA at the end of chromosomes – in people's white blood cells. Telomeres are known to shorten as a person ages.

They found that men and women who were less active tended to have shorter telomeres than those who did plenty of exercise, suggesting that their cells age at a faster rate than active people's cells.

Writing in the *Archives of Internal Medicine*, the study authors said: 'A sedentary lifestyle increases the propensity to ageing-related disease and premature death.

'Inactivity may diminish life expectancy not only by predisposing to ageing-related diseases but also because it may influence the ageing process itself.'

The researchers noted that the link between telomere length and a person's level of physical activity during leisure time was apparent even after body mass index, smoking, socioeconomic status and level of physical activity at work had been taken into account.

They revealed: 'The mean difference in leukocyte (white blood cells) telomere length between the most active [who performed an average of 199 minutes of physical activity per week] and least active [16 minutes of physical activity per week] subjects was 200 nucleotides, which means that the most active subjects had telomeres the same length as sedentary individuals up to ten years younger, on average.'

Exactly how lack of exercise affects telomere length is yet to be unravelled, but the researchers said that the results highlight the importance of regular exercise.

'They show that adults who partake in regular physical activity are biologically younger than sedentary individuals. This conclusion provides a powerful message that could be used by clinicians to promote the potential anti-ageing effect of regular exercise,' they concluded.

News provided by Adfero in collaboration with Cancer Research UK. Please note that all copy is © Adfero Ltd and does not reflect the views or opinions of Cancer Research UK unless explicitly stated.

30 January 2008

⇨ www.cancerresearchuk.org. This information is reprinted with kind permission from Cancer Research UK and Adfero.

© Adfero

Childhood obesity: a class and a classroom issue

Information from the Economic and Social Research Council

By Pamela Readhead

Rising levels of childhood obesity have become both a serious health and social issue. The solutions, on the face of it, are straightforward – more exercise and better diets for children. In devising prescriptions, however, society needs to be aware of the more complex explanations for the rise in obesity, to do with both class and gender, as Pamela Readhead explains.

These days we're bombarded with judgemental media stories about fat kids and their parents, so much so that earlier this year the *Sun* invited its readers to contact the paper if they knew anyone more obese than an 11-year-old boy who weighed 14 stone.

The facts make grim reading. In September Ed Balls, the Secretary of State for Children, Schools and Families, warned that almost half of all children in Britain will be dangerously overweight by 2050 if drastic action is not taken to halt the growth in childhood obesity.

To make matters worse, a study of over 5,500 children at the University of Bath found that children are not taking enough exercise. The research, which was part of the Children of the 90s study, found that only five per cent of boys and 0.4 per cent of girls achieved the recommended minimum of one hour of physical activity per day.

The World Health Organisation (WHO) says this is not just a UK problem. According to the WHO, 20 per cent of children across Europe are overweight, their ranks swelling by 400,000 a year. More worryingly, the world's largest chronic health problem is not HIV/Aids but obesity. More people are overweight (1 billion) than starving (800 million).

Attempts to encourage adults to adopt healthy habits have so far had limited success and the Government now hopes that targeting children will be more effective. Since the beginning of the new term schools in England have banned the sale of all chocolate bars, flavoured biscuits, sweets, crisps and cereal bars in the tuck shop. Salt will no longer be provided on tables, ketchup and mayonnaise will be limited and cakes will be allowed at lunchtime only. New restrictions on junk food and drink radio ads aimed at pre-school and primary school children have also come into force.

> **Society needs to be aware of the more complex explanations for the rise in obesity, to do with both class and gender**

Children are also being encouraged to exercise more. About 80 per cent of secondary school children now do two hours of sport a week – 30 per cent more than in 2003-04. By 2008, the Government wants to see 85 per cent of secondary school pupils doing that much, and by 2020 all those at secondary school should be offered four hours of sport every week.

Social science is also trying to tackle the obesity problem, from several different perspectives. Is obesity related to social class? Why do girls give up on sport? How have children's eating patterns changed since 1975? These are some of the questions that have been addressed by ESRC researchers.

Dr Wendy Wills at the University of Hertfordshire, who is looking at the relationship between attitudes to food and social class, has found a sharp contrast in attitudes and behaviour relating to food amongst two groups of Scottish teenagers and their families. Her joint study with Professor Kathryn Backett-Milburn, Dr Julia Lawton and Dr Donna MacKinnon at the University of Edinburgh suggests that the way of life of the middle-class families bears few similarities with the working-class

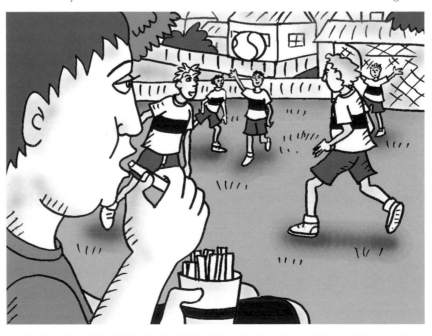

families interviewed for an earlier study. 'It sounds obvious,' she says, 'but when you see the differences in black and white it's no wonder there are health inequalities. Advice on healthy eating will never work for certain groups unless we can understand these differences.'

These days we're bombarded with judgemental media stories about fat kids and their parents

---

The results of the study are still being analysed, but the early findings suggest that the middle-class families make a point of buying fruit and vegetables and worry if their teenagers don't eat a wide variety of different foods. 'The teenagers mentioned foods like Thai curries,' Dr Wills explains. 'This is so different from the first group where the staple diet is far more limited, with an emphasis on ready meals, pot noodles and deep fried takeaways. Policy needs to take account of class habits – or social context – which is so ingrained we all take it for granted, rarely going beyond the boundaries of our own experience. Food culture is part of who we are.'

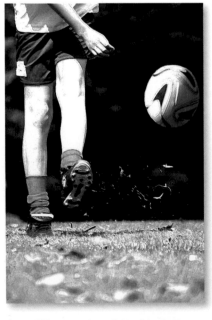

Will more exercise and better diets solve the escalating childhood obesity problem?

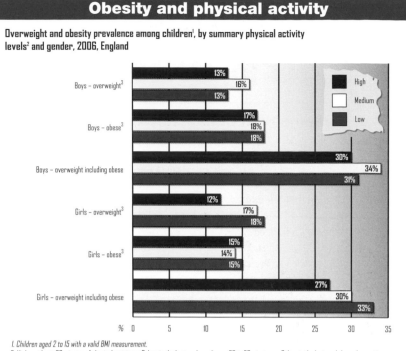

Obesity and physical activity

Overweight and obesity prevalence among children[1], by summary physical activity levels[2] and gender, 2006, England

Legend: High / Medium / Low

- Boys – overweight[3]: 13%, 16%, 13%
- Boys – obese[3]: 17%, 18%, 18%
- Boys – overweight including obese: 30%, 34%, 31%
- Girls – overweight[3]: 12%, 17%, 18%
- Girls – obese[3]: 15%, 14%, 15%
- Girls – overweight including obese: 27%, 30%, 33%

% 0   5   10   15   20   25   30   35

1. Children aged 2 to 15 with a valid BMI measurement.
2. High = at least 60 minutes of physical activity on 7 days in the last week; medium = 30 to 59 minutes on 7 days in the last week; low = less active.
3. Categories are independent, i.e. overweight does not include those who are obese. Overweight was defined as ≥ 85th < 95th UK BMI percentile; obese was defined as ≥ 95th UK BMI percentile.

Source: Health Survey for England 2006. The Information Centre 2008.

Other findings, which are based on interviews with a group of 36 boys and girls aged 13-15 years defined by their BMI as obese/overweight or non-obese/overweight, suggest that middle-class teenagers and their parents are aware of health messages, although they seldom discussed medical problems like diabetes. 'The working-class parents talked about health much more often, but seemed not to be aware that there was a connection between heart problems and diet,' she says. 'They were more concerned about the health consequences of smoking and drug taking and the possibility of anorexia than the dangers of obesity.'

Paola De Agostini at the ESRC Centre on Micro-social Change at the University of Essex has found evidence that young people are consuming much more fat than their parents did at the same age. Paola studied data from the National Food Survey to find out how eating habits changed over a 25-year period. She found that although total calorie intake did not change much across generations between 1975 and 2000, the tendency was for people of all ages to consume more fat and fewer carbohydrates. This was particularly marked for adolescents, probably because they tend to eat out more often, the report says.

In her study of tomboys, Professor Carrie Paechter at the University of London's Goldsmiths College, followed two groups of 9- to 11-year-old girls in contrasting schools as they moved from year five into year six. 'In year five, most of the girls are still running around. But by the time they get into year six they have stopped moving and stand around and chat,' the research says.

So what stops girls from being active? The researchers found that popularity plays a big part. Another reason is clothes. The study concludes that simple policy changes could encourage girls to stay active longer. 'Every school should allow girls to wear trousers and all children to wear trainers and space could be reserved for girls' games to stop the boys from taking over the playground,' the report says.

Autumn 2007

⇨ The above information is re-printed with kind permission from the Economic and Social Research Council, and is taken from the Autumn 2007 issue of their publication *The Edge*. Visit www.esrcsocietytoday. ac.uk for more information.

© ESRC

Eleven-year-olds not taking enough exercise

Information from the University of Bristol

Less than three per cent of UK 11-year-olds are taking enough exercise, suggests research published ahead of print in the *Archives of Disease in Childhood*.

It is recommended that kids spend at least an hour a day doing some form of moderate to vigorous physical activity, in a bid to promote good health and stave off the risks of subsequent obesity and diabetes.

The researchers monitored the physical activity levels of more than 5,500 11-year-olds in the south-west of England over seven consecutive days between January 2003 and January 2005.

The children were part of the Avon Longitudinal Study of Parents and Children (ALSPAC), which has tracked the health of more than 14,000 children since birth.

Each child was kitted out with a special piece of equipment (accelerometer), worn on an elasticated belt, which recorded minute by minute the intensity and frequency of physical activity.

The researchers were particularly interested in total levels of physical activity and the amount of moderate to vigorous exercise the kids were taking daily.

When the data were analysed, they showed that the children were around twice as physically active as adults, but they were still not active enough.

Boys were more physically active than girls, and they were also more likely to engage in moderate to vigorous forms of activity.

One in five (22 per cent) girls averaged at least one bout of moderate to vigorous activity a day, lasting at least five minutes. This compares with 40 per cent of the boys.

But both sexes spent most of their day in light intensity activities. Less than one per cent of the children averaged at least one 20-minute bout a day.

And only just over five per cent of the boys and 0.4 per cent of the girls actually achieved current recommended daily levels of physical activity, equating to 2.5 per cent across both sexes.

Only sustained activity is likely to promote cardiorespiratory fitness, say the authors, adding: 'It is a sobering thought that children's activity levels actually peak at around this age [11] and decline precipitously during adolescence.'

Objective measurement of levels and patterns of physical activity, Online First Arch Dis Child 2007; doi: 10.1136/adc.2006.112136.
13 September 2007

⇨ The above information is reprinted with kind permission from the University of Bristol and was published by the Children of the 90s project. Visit www.bristol.ac.uk for more information.

© University of Bristol

Persecuting chubby kids

The obesity scare is zapping the fun out of childhood and giving rise to the state-sponsored persecution of fat children

By Brendan O'Neill

The childhood obesity scare has gone too far – way too far. It is zapping the fun out of childhood, screwing up children's attitudes to food, and potentially giving rise to a new round of anti-fat kid persecution in the nation's playgrounds.

Earlier this week, the Food Standards Agency declared that two-year-olds should be eating fewer fatty foods – two-year-olds! 'Even toddlers could reduce fats', screamed the headlines. Today, Jessica Mitchell reports on Cif that the Associate Parliamentary Food and Health Forum has concluded its year-long inquiry into the influence of nutrition on mental health (public money well spent, I'm sure): it has recommended that artificial colours and non-essential preservatives be prohibited from food products and soft drinks because apparently they make children hyperactive. So, kids, if nice food doesn't make you fat, it might make you temporarily deranged.

Some schools have already outlawed sweets, crisps, chocolate, chips, salt and anything else that looks, tastes or smells tantalising to young people. Such is the strength of officialdom's jihad against junk food that, as I reported for the BBC in 2006, in some schools entrepreneurial students are smuggling in sweets in order to sell them in a new playground-based black market of contraband confectionery. In other schools, teachers and dinner ladies now rifle through kids' lunchboxes and send a stern letter home to mum and dad if they fail to provide government-approved (or at least Jamie Oliver-approved) healthy grub.

Ed Balls, secretary of state for children, schools and families, is introducing compulsory cookery lessons in September for those between 11 and 14 years old. They won't be like Home Economics lessons of old, where we made rubbish cakes, chucked dough at some pupils and flirted with others, and learnt a few social skills; instead compulsory cooking is being institutionalised because 'teaching kids to cook healthy meals is an important way schools can help produce healthy adults'. In short, children will be inculcated with the government's soulless message about food-as-morality.

Worst of all, the government has proposed weighing schoolchildren as young as four to determine whether they have an acceptable Body Mass Index. Where old racist regimes measured children's facial features to ensure they were properly Aryan, the health-obsessed New Labour regime wants to measure kids' height, weight and waistlines to make sure they are morally-upstanding citizens-to-be who have resisted the temptation to gorge on evil junk food.

Researchers at Loughborough University have expressed concern that such humiliating tests of pupils' BMI could lead to children being 'misinformed about the state of their health and being bullied'. Perfectly healthy and happy children who happen to have a bit of puppy fat or boyish chubbiness could fall foul of the authorities' tyrannical weight-monitoring regime. The Loughborough researchers are worried that we might end up with the degrading practice of 'fat laps'

in the UK: this is when overweight children are made to run off their excess weight, sometimes in full view of other, jeering children. They have already been reported in Australia, where there's a childhood obesity panic similar to ours.

The government has proposed weighing schoolchildren as young as four to determine whether they have an acceptable Body Mass Index

---

The obesity panic is potentially doing far more damage to children – on physical, emotional and psychological levels – than eating the occasional turkey twizzler or swigging from a bottle of fizzy pop could ever do. It has turned eating sweets, that childhood pleasure which all of the killjoys in the anti-obesity industry enjoyed, into something shameful, a dirty, secretive practice to be carried out behind the bike sheds or in the school loo.

It is making children unnecessarily nervous about what they eat, and depressingly obsessed with getting a bit fat. Jeya Henry, Professor of Human Nutrition at Oxford Brookes University, worked on a study of food and health in a primary school and met a six-year-old boy who tearfully complained about having 'fat thighs'.

'That is sad, isn't it? Terrible,' says Professor Henry. 'Childhood should be a time to enjoy and experiment with food.' Not any more, it seems.

And the obesity panic is no doubt making those kids who are genuinely fat feel more isolated than ever before. In the past, bullied fat kids could turn to teachers, most of whom would say something sensible like: 'There's nothing wrong with being fat, so leave Johnny alone.' How could a teacher say that with a straight face today, when the school system – from the classroom to the lunch hall – is being reoriented around the message that obesity is disgusting and must be wiped out? Fat kids could become the victims of a renewed, virtually state-sponsored fat-bashing in the school's playground.

Dr Michael Fitzpatrick, author of *The Tyranny of Health* and a contributor to spiked, my online magazine, says healthy eating has become 'the highest form of ethical virtue recognised in contemporary society'. What we eat has formed the basis of a new, pernicious moral divide. Those who eat microwave meals, cheap chicken from Tesco and crisps (and we know who they mean) are looked upon as vulgar and self-destructive; those who eat fresh organic produce, free-range chicken and handcooked Kettle chips (and we know who these people are, too) are seen as good, aware, caring, morally superior.

Recently, for an article I was writing, I had cause to venture on to some of those unsavoury pro-anorexia websites. The two most commonly expressed sentiments by the sites' users is that food is somehow a poison and that 'Fat is the Enemy'. In an age when often unfounded food scares are rife – covering everything from additives to E numbers – and when obesity is considered to be public enemy number one, I wonder where these sad, lonely celebrators of anorexia got their ideas from? Perhaps it is not the skinny models in *Vogue* that are making young people screwed up about food, but the top-down state-sponsored war on anything that looks or feels like a bit of puppy fat.
8 February 2008
© Guardian Newspapers Limited 2008

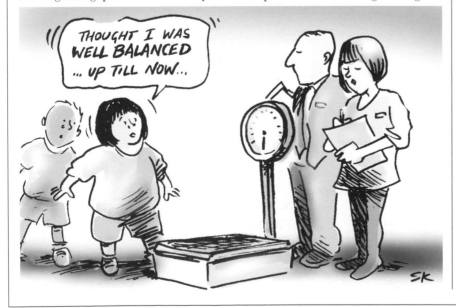

The fitness strategy

Government announces first steps in strategy to help people maintain healthy weight and live healthier lives. Extra £372 million increases opportunity for all to make healthier choices

A new £372 million cross-government strategy to help everyone lead healthier lives was published today by the Health Secretary, Alan Johnson, and the Secretary of State for Children, Schools and Families, Ed Balls.

The Government's groundbreaking strategy supports the creation of a healthy society – from early years, to schools and food, from sport and physical activity to planning, transport and the health service.

Having been at least 30 years in the making, the obesity trend will not be halted overnight

It will bring together employers, individuals and communities to promote children's health and healthy food; build physical activity into our lives; support health at work; and provide incentives more widely to promote health. It will also provide effective treatment and support when people become overweight or obese.

Having been at least 30 years in the making, the obesity trend will not be halted overnight. This strategy is a first step and will be followed by an annual report that assesses progress, looks at the latest evidence and trends and makes recommendations for further action. A panel of experts will assist the Government, with input from a new public health obesity observatory that will develop our understanding of what changes behaviour.

Alan Johnson said:

'Tackling obesity is the most significant public and personal health challenge facing our society. The core of the problem is simple – we eat too much and we do too little exercise. The solution is more complex. From the nature of the food that we eat, to the built environment, through to the way our children lead their lives – it is harder to avoid obesity in the modern environment.

'It is not the Government's role to hector or lecture people, but we do have a duty to support them in leading healthier lifestyles. This will only succeed if the problem is recognised, owned and addressed in every part of society.'

The five key elements of the strategy are:

First, the healthy growth and development of children.

⇨ Early identification of at-risk families and plans to make breastfeeding the default option for mothers.

⇨ Investment in healthy schools, increasing participation in physical activity, and making cooking a compulsory part of the national curriculum.

⇨ A £75 million marketing campaign to support and empower parents to make changes to their children's diet and increase levels of physical activity.

Second, promoting healthier food choices.

⇨ Setting out a Healthy Food Code of Good Practice to be finalised in partnership with the food and drink industry, including proposals to develop a single, simple and effective approach to food labelling, and to challenge the industry (including restaurants and food outlets) to support individuals and families reduce their consumption of saturated fat, salt and sugar.

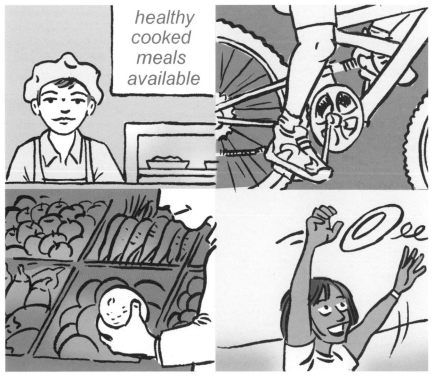

healthy cooked meals available

⇨ OFCOM to bring forward its review of the restrictions already introduced on the advertising of unhealthy foods to children.

⇨ Promote Local Authority planning powers to limit the spread of fast food outlets in particular areas e.g. such as close to schools or parks.

Third, building physical activity into our lives.

⇨ Investment of £30 million in 'Healthy Towns' – working with selected towns and cities to bring together the successful EPODE (Ensemble Prevenons Lobesite Des Enfants) model used in Europe, using infrastructure and whole town approaches to promoting physical activity.

⇨ Set up a working group with the entertainment technology industry to ensure that they continue to develop tools to allow parents to manage the time that their children spend watching TV or playing sedentary games, online and much more widely.

⇨ Review our overall approach to physical activity, including the role of Sport England, with the aim of producing a fresh set of programmes to ensure that there is a clear legacy of increased physical activity before and after the 2012 Games.

Fourth, creating incentives for better health.

⇨ Stronger incentives for individuals, employers and the NHS to prioritise the long-term work of improving health.

⇨ Working with employers and employer organisations to explore how companies can best promote good health among their staff and make healthy workplaces part of their core business model.

⇨ We will pilot and evaluate a range of different approaches to using personal financial incentives to encourage healthy living.

Fifth, personalised advice and support.

⇨ Developing the NHS Choices website so that it provides advice for diet and activity levels, with clear and consistent information on how to maintain a healthy weight.

⇨ Increased funding over the next three years to support the commissioning of more weight management services, where people can access personalised services to support them in achieving real and sustained weight loss.

'Every parent wants their child to be fit and healthy – what we want to do is help them make informed decisions about their own children's lives'

In England alone, nearly a quarter of men and women are now obese. The trends for children are even more cause for concern, with 18 per cent of 2- to 15-year-olds currently obese and a further 14 per cent overweight.

The Foresight report on obesity, published last year, indicated that on current trends nearly 60 per cent of the UK population will be obese by 2050 – that is almost two out of three in the population defined as severely overweight. If this trend continues, millions of adults and children will inevitably face deteriorating health and a lower quality of life and we face spiralling health and social care costs.

Ed Balls said:

'Tackling obesity in the adults of tomorrow requires winning the hearts and minds of young people today.

'Every parent wants their child to be fit and healthy – what we want to do is help them make informed decisions about their own children's lives.

'And giving young people the lifelong education they need – more sport and exercise in and out of school; ending the "no ball games" culture with more play and sports facilities; equipping children with cooking skills and understanding of diet; and stamping out unhealthy and junk food in schools.'

The Chief Medical Officer, Sir Liam Donaldson, said:

'This cross-government strategy on obesity has come at a vitally important time. It has never been more challenging to maintain a healthy weight as it is today. A unified solution must be found and this is an important first stage in engaging the whole of society in this issue. As mentioned in my annual report of 2002, physical activity, healthy eating, balanced marketing and promotion of food to children and clear and consistent food labelling are all key components in beating the obesity time bomb.'

23 January 2008

⇨ The above information is re-printed with kind permission from the Department of Health. Visit www.dh.gov.uk for more information.

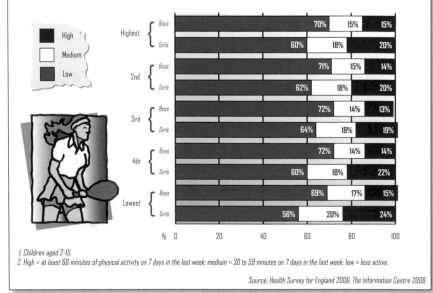

Physical activity and income

Children's physical activity levels[2], by equivalised household income and gender, 2006, England

		High	Medium	Low
Highest	Boys	70%	15%	15%
	Girls	60%	18%	20%
2nd	Boys	71%	15%	14%
	Girls	62%	18%	20%
3rd	Boys	72%	14%	13%
	Girls	64%	18%	19%
4th	Boys	72%	14%	14%
	Girls	60%	18%	22%
Lowest	Boys	69%	17%	15%
	Girls	56%	20%	24%

% 0   20   40   60   80   100

1. Children aged 2-15.
2. High = at least 60 minutes of physical activity on 7 days in the last week; medium = 30 to 59 minutes on 7 days in the last week; low = less active.

Source: Health Survey for England 2006. The Information Centre 2008.

Tackling obesities: future choices

Summary of key messages from the Foresight
Tackling Obesities: Future Choices report

By looking ahead 40 years, using scientific evidence, commissioned research and expert advice, the Foresight project, *Tackling Obesities: Future Choices* has taken a strategic view of the issue of obesity.

By 2050, Foresight modelling indicates that 60% of adult men, 50% of adult women and about 25% of all children under 16 could be obese

---

In recent years Britain has become a nation where overweight is the norm. The rate of increase in overweight and obesity, in children and adults, is striking. By 2050, Foresight modelling indicates that 60% of adult men, 50% of adult women and about 25% of all children under 16 could be obese. Obesity increases the risk of a range of chronic diseases, particularly type 2 diabetes, stroke and coronary heart disease and also cancer and arthritis. The NHS costs attributable to overweight and obesity are projected to double to £10 billion per year by 2050. The wider costs to society and business are estimated to reach £49.9 billion per year (at today's prices).

The causes of obesity are extremely complex encompassing biology and behaviour, but set within a cultural, environmental and social framework. There is compelling evidence that humans are predisposed to put on weight by their biology. This has previously been concealed in all but a few but exposure to modern lifestyles has revealed it in the majority. Although personal responsibility plays a crucial part in weight gain, human biology is being overwhelmed by the effects of today's 'obesogenic' environment, with its abundance of energy dense food, motorised transport and sedentary lifestyles. As a result, the people of the UK are inexorably becoming heavier simply by living in the Britain of today. This process has been coined 'passive obesity'. Some members of the population, including the most disadvantaged, are especially vulnerable to the conditions.

Successfully tackling obesity is a long-term, large-scale commitment. The current prevalence of obesity in the population has been at least 30 years in the making. This will take time to reverse and it will be least 30 years before reductions in the associated diseases are seen. The evidence is very clear that policies aimed solely at individuals will be inadequate and that simply increasing the number or type of small-scale interventions will not be sufficient to reverse this trend. Significant effective action to prevent obesity at a population level is required.

Foresight's work indicates that a bold whole system approach is critical – from production and promotion of healthy diets to redesigning the built environment to promote walking, together with wider cultural changes to shift societal values around food and activity. This will require a broad set of integrated policies including both population and targeted measures and must necessarily include action not only by government, both central and local, but also action by industry, communities, families and society as a whole.

Tackling obesity has striking similarities with tackling climate change. Both need whole societal change with cross-governmental action and long-term commitment. Many climate-change goals would also help prevent obesity, such as measures to reduce traffic congestion, increase cycling or design sustainable communities. Tackling them together would enhance the effectiveness of action. There are also synergies with other policy goals such as increasing social inclusion and narrowing health inequalities since obesity's impact is greatest on the poorest. No other country yet has an integrated, whole system approach to the prevention of obesity. Yet, based on the UK's strengths in research, surveillance and public health, there is an opportunity to pioneer a new approach that sets the global standards for success.

October 2007

⇨ The above information is reprinted with kind permission from Foresight, the government office for science. Visit www.foresight.gov.uk for more information.

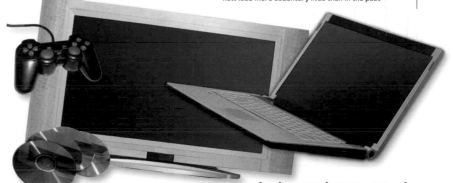

The prevalence of home technology is one reason why we now lead more sedentary lives than in the past

Surgery and drugs not enough to combat obesity

Information from the University of Bristol

A review of research examining the effectiveness of different obesity treatments has concluded that no matter what other forms of therapy are offered, changes in lifestyle are imperative if patients want to maximise and maintain their weight loss.

The results, presented at the annual Society for Endocrinology BES meeting in Harrogate, show that lifestyle interventions provide benefits at all stages of obesity management and should be encouraged, no matter what other forms of therapy are offered.

Dr Rob Andrews from the University of Bristol carried out a review of the research on weight loss methods published in international peer-reviewed journals. He examined how successful different lifestyle interventions (such as exercise, diet and behavioural therapies) are in the treatment of obesity when carried out alone or in combination with other treatments such as surgery to cause weight loss (bariatric surgery) and weight loss drugs.

Dr Rob Andrews said: 'People often forget is that there is no quick fix to obesity. Overeating and decreased activity are the fundamental problems underlying the development of obesity. Any therapy aimed at helping obese patients must have a dietary and exercise component in order to be successful. This review shows that patients who are taking weight loss drugs or have bariatric surgery lose significantly more weight if they combine these treatments with regular exercise and a calorie-controlled diet. Maintaining a healthy, balanced lifestyle is the key to maximising and maintaining weight loss.'

Andrews found that when weight loss drugs are given on their own, with no other changes in lifestyle, they produce an average weight loss of 5kg, the same amount of weight you lose if you go on a calorie-controlled diet and take regular exercise. However, if weight loss drugs are offered in combination with behavioural therapies, their effectiveness can be increased by over 100% (from 5kg to 12kg average weight loss).

The story was the same with bariatric surgery. Patients who exercise and lose weight prior to surgery are less likely to have postoperative complications and lose more weight at a quicker rate after surgery than those who did not.

Overall, this review indicates that when treating obese patients, weight loss drugs and bariatric surgery are significantly more successful if they are offered in conjunction with improvements to diet and exercise.

Full results of the review are:

⇨ Exercise alone produces an average weight loss of 1.8kg. The more you exercise the more weight you lose.

⇨ Diet alone produces an average weight loss of 5.0kg. This effect peaks 6-12 months following the start of the diet and wanes after this point. No diet is better than any other in the long term but the greater the reduction in calories, the greater the initial weight loss.

⇨ Behavioural therapies (e.g. cognitive therapy, psychotherapy, relaxation therapy, hypnotherapy) produce an average weight loss of 2.3kg.

⇨ Exercise plus diet results in an average weight loss of 10.7kg and helps to maintain weight loss for a longer period.

⇨ Exercise plus diet plus behavioural therapies results in the greatest average weight loss of 12-15kg.

⇨ Taking weight loss drugs with no changes in lifestyle results in an average weight loss of 5kg. Taking weight loss drugs, in combination with behavioural therapies, leads to an average weight loss of 12kg.

⇨ Patients that lose more than 10% of their body weight prior to bariatric surgery are 2.12 times more likely to achieve a 70% loss of excess body weight.

10 April 2008

⇨ The above information is reprinted with kind permission from the University of Bristol. Visit www.bristol.ac.uk for more information.

© *University of Bristol*

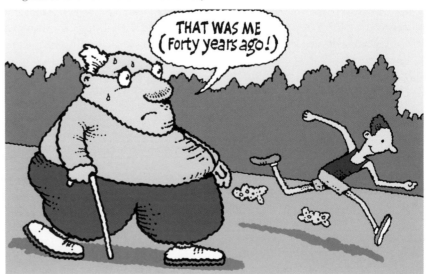

THAT WAS ME (Forty years ago!)

Obesity discrimination

Government comes under pressure to make discrimination against obese people illegal. By Karen Dempsey

The government is coming under increasing pressure to make 'fattism' unlawful after The Obesity Awareness & Solutions Trust (TOAST) stepped up its efforts to make tackling obesity a national health priority.

The charity has been drumming up support among MPs to press for action on obesity, which costs the economy up to £3.7bn and accounts for 18 million sick days per year, according to a Commons committee on obesity.

Dr Brian Iddon, Labour MP for Bolton South East, and a patron of TOAST, suggested the government should consider making it illegal to discriminate against people because of their size.

'This government has gone to great lengths in its efforts to abolish discrimination in several areas of social policy. Obviously, it will have to look next at discrimination against those who are overweight,' he said.

Louise Diss, the charity's chief executive, added: 'Anti-discrimination legislation is part of the solution, but it won't stop people getting fat. It's not just about a change in the law it's about discussing how to deal with it.'

This move comes as we reveal the findings of our obesity awareness survey, carried out among 2,603 readers of *Personnel Today*, and 331 members of TOAST.

An astonishing 93% of HR professionals said there was a social stigma about obesity, yet two-thirds admitted the issue was not discussed enough in their organisation. Almost three-quarters said their organisation was not actively tackling obesity, and only one-third ensured that managers were vigilant for any teasing or bullying.

Yet the TOAST members who responded believed that employers were more likely to select obese workers for redundancy or pass them over for promotion, and were not sympathetic to obese staff.

When we last carried out this survey in October 2005, 93% of HR professionals said they would hire a 'normal weight' candidate rather than an obese one who was identically qualified. Nothing has changed since then: our new survey reveals that 93% would still make that choice.

TV personality Anne Diamond, who runs Fathappens.com, said obesity should be 'the new smoking'. 'HR and bosses should blaze the trail,' she said. 'This current attitude to fat has got to stop.'

Feedback from the profession

⇨ David Bornor, head of HR, The Children's Mutual: 'I don't believe good employers will discriminate on grounds of obesity. The stigma is more about visual aesthetics. Employers can only do so much: they should try not to make things worse, but it is down to the individual to address this issue.'

⇨ Andrew Marston, assistant chief officer (HR), Greater Manchester Police: 'I don't think you can have a policy on obesity, but HR professionals need to be alive to the issues and have some proactive strategies in place.'

⇨ Cara Davani, group director corporate services, Genesis Housing Group: 'Appearance is critical to establishing credibility in an interview situation, but it does not mean that obese people cannot be well presented. This survey shows the importance of including access to information and advice on healthy lifestyles and diet in a health promotions programme. Ultimately, the employer and employee have shared responsibilities for health in the workplace.'

⇨ Stephen Hall, vice-president, HR, Metronet Rail: 'Obesity has always been the "unspoken problem", particularly with regard to recruitment. But selection for redundancy on grounds of obesity is a real myth.'

13 March 2007

⇨ Information from *Personnel Today*. Visit www.personneltoday.com

© *Personnel Today*

Obesity in the workplace

Results of independent market research from Nuffield

⇨ 68% of employers believe obesity is a serious issue in the workplace contributing to lower productivity and higher costs.

⇨ The majority of employers (60%) believe that employees who are obese are more likely to have time off sick than those who are not.

⇨ 91% of employers believe that obese people are at a disadvantage in the job market.

⇨ Nearly three-quarters of employers (72%) think that obesity can be perceived as a reflection of negative characteristics in an employee (such as laziness or lack of self-control) even though they may not express this openly.

⇨ 9 out of 10 employers who would like to talk to obese staff about their health feel reluctant to do so due to concerns about the person's feelings and/or possible legal implications.

⇨ Only 2% of organisations offer support and/or advice for employees concerned about their weight, with only 5% planning to do anything about it in the future.

⇨ The above information is reprinted with kind permission from Nuffield Proactive Health. Visit www.nuffieldproactivehealth.com for more.

© *Nuffield Proactive Health*

Obesity crisis: get paid to lose weight

By Rebecca Smith, Medical Editor

Fat people will be offered cash incentives to lose weight and take regular exercise under a radical Government strategy announced yesterday to tackle the obesity epidemic.

A recent analysis of nine research studies which used financial incentives found there was no effect on weight after 12 months

Employers will be encouraged to set up competitions with money, vouchers and other rewards for people who give up junk food in favour of healthy eating and living. Those losing the most weight would earn the biggest prizes.

Ministers believe that by giving people incentives to do something about their weight now, it will help avoid larger costs associated with treating cancer, heart disease and diabetes caused by obesity. Similar schemes have worked well in America and British medical insurance companies already offer discounts for people who go to the gym regularly.

Experts say that most of the population will be obese by 2050 unless urgent action is taken and the associated rise in ill health would cost the NHS £50 billion a year.

The Government wants Britain to be the first major nation to reverse the rising tide of obesity and said it would focus on reducing within 12 years the proportion of children who are overweight back to the 2000 level of 26 per cent.

At present, 30 per cent of children are obese or overweight.

The Government said schools should consider banning children from going out of the gates at lunchtime and town councils are being urged to block new fast food outlets near parks and schools.

Yesterday's milestone strategy – Healthy Weight, Healthy Lives – highlighted a series of projects run through the Well@Work scheme, led by the British Heart Foundation, which offer rewards for workers who lose weight.

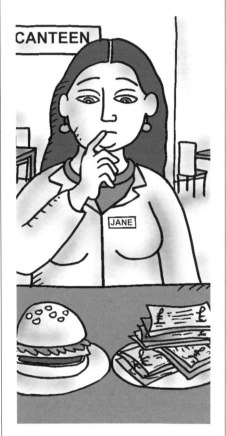

One competition, called The Biggest Loser, awarded £130 in gift vouchers for the participant who lost the most weight. Ministers want to encourage more such schemes in the workplace.

The strategy said: 'We will look at using financial incentives, such as payments, vouchers and other rewards, to encourage individuals to lose weight and sustain that weight loss, to eat more healthily, or to be consistently more physically active.'

It is not clear from the strategy who would fund such schemes but the onus is likely to be on companies as they could expect to benefit from

Key points

⇨ Individual and company incentives to encourage a healthier lifestyle with payments, vouchers for leisure centres under consideration.

⇨ New target to reduce childhood obesity to the levels of 2000. The present rate is 30 per cent and rising each year.

⇨ Compulsory cooking lessons in secondary schools by 2011 and healthy packed lunch policies in all schools.

⇨ A £75 million marketing campaign to inform parents of the importance of a healthy diet and physical activity.

⇨ £140 million to improve cycling facilities for children in areas where childhood obesity is a particular problem.

⇨ The NHS Choices website to develop personalised advice services on diet and activity.

⇨ More NHS weight management programmes to be commissioned.

⇨ Promotion to make breastfeeding the norm with a national helpline and a code of practice for employers.

⇨ Development of a single food labelling system to be used by all supermarkets.

⇨ £30m for healthy towns projects where walking, cycling, parks and use of stairs instead of lifts is incorporated into buildings and the environment.

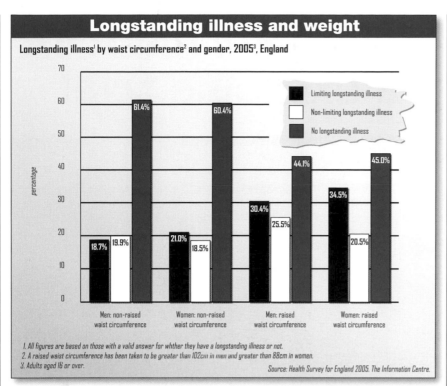

Longstanding illness and weight

Longstanding illness[1] by waist circumference[2] and gender, 2005[3], England

Legend:
- Limiting longstanding illness
- Non-limiting longstanding illness
- No longstanding illness

Men: non-raised waist circumference — 18.7%, 19.9%, 61.4%
Women: non-raised waist circumference — 21.0%, 18.5%, 60.4%
Men: raised waist circumference — 30.4%, 25.5%, 44.1%
Women: raised waist circumference — 34.5%, 20.5%, 45.0%

percentage (y-axis 0–70)

1. All figures are based on those with a valid answer for whther they have a longstanding illness or not.
2. A raised waist circumference has been taken to be greater than 102cm in men and greater than 88cm in women.
3. Adults aged 16 or over.

Source: Health Survey for England 2005. The Information Centre.

a healthier workforce. It is likely that the schemes would also be tax deductible.

The Government is investing £372 million over three years to implement the strategy and annual progress reports will be published.

more fruit and vegetables was more effective than paying for weight loss.

Andrew Lansley, the shadow health secretary, accused the Government of stealing his party's ideas for healthy lifestyle reward vouchers, but criticised plans for cash handouts for shedding pounds.

However, Dr Ian Campbell, the medical director of Weight Concern, said work-based incentive schemes were a 'win win' because the employer benefited from a workforce that was less likely to take time off sick, while employees improved their health.

He said: 'It might sound a bit desperate but we are desperate so we have to look at all these things.'

A spokesman for the Department of Health said: 'The use of incentives is at a very early stage. We are working with the experts, looking at the success of schemes worldwide that have been used in the public and private sector.'

A person with a Body Mass Index (BMI) of 25 is overweight, those with a BMI above 30 are classed as obese. A healthy BMI is between 18.5 and 25.

BMI is calculated by dividing weight in kilograms by height in metres squared. A BMI of 20 to 25 is considered normal, 25 to 30 overweight, and over 30 obese.

28 January 2008

© *Telegraph Group Limited, London 2008*

Experts say that most of the population will be obese by 2050 unless urgent action is taken and the associated rise in ill health would cost the NHS £50 billion a year

---

Dr David Haslam, the clinical director of the National Obesity Forum, said the incentives scheme smacked of 'desperation'. There was little evidence that payments would work and it would be difficult to check whether people were regularly taking exercise.

A recent analysis of nine research studies which used financial incentives found there was no effect on weight after 12 months. Aberdeen University's Health Services Research Unit said eating

Make all staff exercise for an hour, says health adviser

By Georgina Littlejohn

A radical plan to improve the nation's health – including a workplace 'exercise hour' – has been unveiled by a leading Government adviser.

New figures today show England is the fattest country in the EU. Now Professor Julian Le Grand, chairman of Health England, hopes to encourage people to improve their diets, give up smoking and exercise more.

He proposed the introduction of a smoking permit, which smokers would be required to show each time they bought tobacco. It is then their choice to go smoke free and not buy a permit.

Companies with more than 500 staff would have an 'exercise hour'. Employees would have to deliberately choose not to join in. The proposals are the opposite of the Government's approach which requires people to opt in to healthy lifestyles. Instead it would be up to them to make the unhealthy choice.

In his speech to the Royal Statistical Society last night the professor, a former aide to Tony Blair said: 'It is not like banning something, it's a softer form of paternalism.'

⇨ This article first appeared in the *Evening Standard*, 23 October 2007

© *2008 Associated Newspapers Ltd*

Fitness barriers broken in workplace exercise trial

Information from the University of Leeds

Psychologists from the University of Leeds are helping to motivate more than 1,000 workers to get fit in a work-based study into physical activity and health – believed to be the first of its kind in the UK.

Bus drivers, office staff and managers from three major organisations have signed up to the trial run by a team from the University's Institute of Psychological Sciences in partnership with the Health and Safety Laboratory and funded by a £300,000 grant from the BUPA Foundation.

British business loses 21 million days due to sickness. The North West lost the most days in 2006 at 8.8 days per employee.

Health psychologist Dr Rebecca Lawton, who is leading the team, said: 'Exercise not only reduces the risk of physical illness and therefore sickness absence, but can also lessen anxiety and depression and help people to perform everyday tasks better.'

Dr Lawton's team found people's number one obstacle to being active is time. Now they have developed a toolkit of materials to help people overcome barriers and encourage a change in attitude towards getting fit.

The team recruited employees in sedentary jobs from Wrexham Council, a leading Yorkshire teaching hospital and the Leeds and York depots of transport business FirstGroup, where the trial is also being supported by the UK's largest trade union, Unite.

Dr Lawton said: 'Many of us sit for long periods of the day at work. The organisations we are working with want to give their staff the opportunity to become more active because this has real benefits for health and well-being.

'We hope the trial will help change the way people think about activity and that by working in groups with peer group support our participants and their employers will see real changes.'

The toolkit includes a fridge magnet to help participants monitor their exercise as well as tips and hints to getting fit, such as challenging teams of employees to scale a virtual mountain by climbing stairs.

More than 200 FirstGroup bus drivers from Leeds and York are taking part in the trial. Operations director David Phillips said: 'Our drivers can be behind the wheel for up to 10 hours a day so I believe we have a responsibility as an employer to look after their well-being.

'However, people often don't know where to start, where to go and who to talk to. We see the research as a stepping stone to promoting health and linking with other partners, such as local gyms.'

Wales has the fourth highest number of days lost per employee at 8.1. Wrexham County Borough Council already holds the Gold category in the Welsh Assembly's Corporate Health Standard, designed to recognise employers who encourage and support the health and well-being of their employees. Ten per cent of the council's 6,000 employees are taking part in the trial.

Claire Broad, who works in the council's Prevention and Inclusion Department, said: 'The initiative is a great way of raising awareness among staff of the benefits of becoming more active. As a facilitator in one of the council-selected work sites, I hope that the toolkit will continue to support and motivate staff to exercise beyond the life of the project.'

Dr Andrew Vallance-Owen, deputy chairman of the Bupa Foundation, said:

'Dr Lawton and her colleagues were awarded a specialist themed grant to fund projects which promote health in the workplace.

'This study will look at ways to encourage more physical activity in the workplace. With obesity levels increasing and jobs becoming ever more sedentary we hope that the findings will support ways to improve

Exercise barriers

Researchers found that the top 10 barriers to exercise are:
1. I don't have enough time
2. I'm too tired by the time I get home after work
3. I just can't be bothered
4. There aren't any convenient facilities
5. It is more important for me to relax when I'm not working
6. I have too many other commitments
7. I don't like getting and hot and sweaty
8. It's dangerous to do things on my own
9. I'm too embarrassed
10. My manager and colleagues would frown on me taking a break

The biggest incentive to doing exercise was 'Doing things with other people'.

attitudes to health and well-being that are easily transferable to any workplace in future. We eagerly await the progress of the project.'

Staff from the Health and Safety laboratory, an agency of the Health and Safety Executive, are carrying out health checks on all participants in the trial. In each workplace a number of employees are trained to support and encourage their colleagues using the specially designed toolkit.

The trial will compare changes in behaviour, health and work for employees using the toolkit with a comparable group of employees who are not receiving the same motivational methods.

27 March 2008

⇨ The above information is reprinted with kind permission from the University of Leeds. Visit www.leeds.ac.uk for more information.

© *University of Leeds*

Avoiding childhood obesity

This article is for people who have obese children or want to know more about childhood obesity

Children need lots of energy because they are growing. A varied and nutritious diet is essential for their development. However, like adults, if they take in more energy – in the form of food – than they use up, the extra energy is stored in their bodies as fat.

In the UK an estimated one in four 11- to 15-year-olds are overweight or obese – and the problem is growing every year.

A serious problem

Research shows that obese children are at increased risk from a number of serious health problems more usually seen in adulthood, including hardened and blocked arteries (coronary artery diseases), high blood pressure, and type 2 diabetes. When they grow up, they are more likely to be obese.

This means a higher risk of heart attack and stroke, type 2 diabetes, bowel cancer, and high blood pressure in adulthood. The risk of health problems increases the more overweight a person becomes.

Being overweight as a child can also cause psychological distress. Teasing about their appearance affects a child's confidence and self-esteem, and can lead to isolation and depression.

The number of overweight and obese children in the UK has risen steadily over the past 20 years. The obesity epidemic is now a major health concern.

Why are more children overweight?

Very few children become overweight because of an underlying medical problem. Research indicates that children are more likely to be obese if their parents are obese. It isn't known whether this is because of genetic factors which the child inherits, if it's because families tend to share eating and activity habits, or a combination of them both.

However, it's thought that most children put on excess weight because their lifestyles include an unhealthy diet and a lack of physical activity.

It is certainly easier than ever before for children to become overweight. High-calorie foods, such as fast food and confectionery, are abundant, relatively cheap and heavily promoted, specifically at children.

Exercise is no longer a regular part of everyone's day – some children never walk or cycle to school, or play any kind of sport. It is not unusual for children to spend hours in front of a television or computer. According to the National Diet and Nutrition Survey (2000), 4 out of 10 boys and 6 out of 10 girls do not do the minimum one hour a day of physical activity recommended by the then health education authority.

What is a healthy weight for a child?

You may find it difficult to tell whether your child has temporary 'puppy fat' or is genuinely overweight. In adults, a simple formula (the body mass index, or BMI) is used to work out whether a person is the right weight for their height.

However, BMI alone is not an appropriate measure for children, because they are still growing. Factors such as rate of growth, age and sex, and the BMI of other children of the same age must be taken into account when assessing your child's weight. BMI is best interpreted with the help of your GP, health visitor, practice nurse or dietitian.

Maintaining a healthy weight

In most cases, experts recommend that overweight children should not be encouraged to actually lose weight. Instead they should be encouraged to maintain their weight, so that they gradually 'grow into it' as they get taller.

Children should never be put on a weight loss diet without medical advice as this can affect their growth. Unregulated dieting – particularly in teenage girls – is thought to lead to the development of eating disorders. For more information, see the separate BUPA health factsheets, *Anorexia nervosa* and *Bulimia nervosa*.

There isn't much evidence for the best ways to treat weight problems in children, but research indicates that focusing on making long-term improvements to diet and increasing physical activity may be the effective solution.

Helping children to achieve and maintain a healthy weight involves a threefold approach that encourages them to:
- eat a healthy, well-balanced diet;
- make changes to eating habits;
- increase physical activity – in 2004 the Chief Medical Officer recommended at least 60 minutes of at least moderate physical activity a day for children.

The good news is that it is probably easier to change a child's eating and exercise habits than it is to change an adult's.

A healthy well-balanced diet

If you are concerned about your child's weight, encourage a variety of fresh, nutritious foods in his or her diet.
- Starchy foods which are rich in complex carbohydrates are bulky, relative to the amount of calories they contain. This makes them both filling and nutritious. Sources such as bread, potatoes, pasta, rice and chapatti should provide half the energy in a child's diet.
- Instead of high-fat foods like chocolate, biscuits, cakes and crisps, try healthier alternatives such as fresh fruit, crusty bread or crackers.
- Try to grill or bake foods instead of frying. Burgers, fish fingers and sausages are just as tasty when grilled, but have a lower fat content. Oven chips are lower in fat than fried chips.

- Avoid fizzy drinks that are high in sugar. Substitute them with fresh juices diluted with water or sugar-free alternatives.
- A healthy breakfast of a low-sugar cereal (e.g. wholemeal wheat biscuits) with milk, plus a piece of fruit is a good start to the day.
- Instead of sweets, offer dried fruit or tinned fruit in natural juice. Frozen yoghurt is an alternative to ice cream. Bagels are an alternative to doughnuts.

Changes to eating habits

To achieve lasting effects, the whole family attitudes and habits towards food and exercise need to change.

- Try to set a good example with your own eating habits.
- Provide meals and snacks at regular times to prevent 'grazing' throughout the day.
- Don't allow your children to eat while watching TV or doing homework.
- Make mealtimes an occasion by eating as a family group as often as possible.
- Encourage children to 'listen to their tummies' and eat when they are hungry rather than out of habit.
- Teach children to chew food more slowly and savour the food, as they will feel fuller more quickly and be less likely to overeat at mealtimes.
- Don't keep lots of high-fat, high-sugar snack foods in the house.
- Don't make outings for fast foods part of the weekly routine.
- Try to get your children involved in preparing food as this will make them more aware of what they are eating.

Physical activity

Doctors recommend a gradual increase in physical activity, such as brisk walking, to at least an hour a day.

- Encourage walking to places such as school and the shops, rather than always jumping in the car or bus.
- Suggest going to the park for a kick-around with a football, or a game of rounders, cricket or frisbee.
- Visit a local leisure centre to investigate sports and team activities to get involved in.
- Make exercise into a treat by taking special trips to an adventure play park or an ice skating rink, for example. Involve the whole family in bike rides, swimming and in-line skating.
- When it is safe to do so, teach your child to ride a bike.

Reducing physical inactivity

Physically inactive pastimes such as watching TV or playing computer games should be limited to around two hours a day or an average of 14 hours a week. Encourage children to be selective about what they watch and concentrate only on the programmes they really enjoy.

The emotional factors

Food can take on emotional significance when used to comfort or reward children.

- Don't use food to comfort your child – give attention, hugs and listen.
- Avoid using food as a reward as this can reinforce the idea of food as a source of comfort. Instead of having a fast-food meal to celebrate a good school report, for example, buy a gift, go to the cinema, or have a friend to stay overnight.

Prevention

- Some research suggests that breast-feeding your baby may reduce childhood obesity, although the evidence is not conclusive.
- Other studies indicate that smoking during pregnancy increases the risk of having an overweight child.

Further information

- British Nutrition Foundation www.nutrition.org.uk
- Food Standards Agency www.foodstandards.gov.uk/healthiereating

Sources

- Rise in childhood obesity rates – new statistics from health survey for England. The Information Centre. www.ic.nhs.uk accessed 1 November 2006
- Consequences of childhood obesity. SIGN. www.sign.ac.uk accessed 22 November 2006
- Interventions for preventing obesity in children. The Cochrane library, 2006(4).

- Being big or growing fast: systematic review of size and growth in infancy and later obesity. Baird, J., et al. BMJ 2005, 331:929 www.bmj.com accessed 22 November 2006
- Food promotion and children Action Plan 2005 – The facts. Food Standards Agency www.food.gov.uk accessed 22 November 2006
- Obesity and health. Bandolier. Publication 85.

You may find it difficult to tell whether your child has temporary 'puppy fat' or is genuinely overweight

- Obesity – Background Information – Complications and prognosis. Prodigy Knowledge Guidance. www.prodigy.nhs.uk accessed 22 November 2006
- Reilly, J.J., et al. Early life risk factors for obesity in childhood: cohort study. BMJ 2005; 330: 1357. www.bmj.com
- Management of obesity in children and young people. Scottish Intercollegiate Guidelines Network. www.sign.ac.uk accessed 22 November 2006
- Edmunds, L., E. Waters, and E.J. Elliott. Evidence based paediatrics: Evidence based management of childhood obesity. BMJ 2001; 323:916-919
- Interventions for preventing obesity in children. The Cochrane collaboration. The Cochrane library. www.cochrane.org accessed 22 November 2006
- Li, L., Breast feeding and obesity in childhood: cross sectional study. BMJ 2003. 327: 904-905

February 2007

Treat childhood obesity as act of neglect, say doctors

By Matthew Weaver

Doctors said today that childhood obesity should be treated as an act of neglect by parents as reports claimed that obesity had played a part in 20 child protection cases last year.

A group of GPs from Rotherham, South Yorkshire, has tabled a motion to the BMA's annual meeting later this month opening the way for social workers to step in when children become obese.

The motion says: 'The government should consider childhood obesity in under-12s as neglect by the parents and encourage legal protection for the child and action against those parents.'

> **'The government should consider childhood obesity in under-12s as neglect by the parents and encourage legal protection for the child and action against those parents'**

It raises the prospect of more cases such as that of Conor McCreaddie, the 89kg (14st) eight-year-old from Wallsend, Tyne & Wear, whose mother was told that she would lose custody of the boy unless he lost weight.

Rotherham GP Dr Matt Capehorn put forward the motion to the BMA meeting as a result of his own experience of running an obesity clinic.

He told the BBC: 'My colleagues and I were concerned because we noticed a discrepancy in the way society, the medical profession and the courts treat an obese child compared with a malnourished child.

'There is outrage if a child is skin and bone but it only happens in extreme cases with obese children.'

Last year, at least 20 care orders were given for children where obesity was a factor.

One doctor spoke of a 10-year-old girl who could walk only a few yards with a stick. He believed her parents were 'killing her slowly' with a diet of chips and high fat food.

Dr Tabitha Randell, a consultant paediatrician from Nottingham, said she believed some parents were killing their children with kindness.

In one extreme case, she saw a child aged two-and-a-half, who weighed more than 25.4kg (4st).

She said: 'They said she was big boned and they were, too. I think the perception of parents is a very real problem.

'If you see every other child in the playground with their belly hanging over their trousers, you think that's normal.'

But the Royal College of Paediatrics and Child Health expressed caution and said using care orders in these circumstances would be very rare.

Dr Penny Gibson, advisor on childhood obesity for the college, said: 'I think that would be an extremely unusual situation and would be in the context of parents who did not understand the seriousness of the situation and what needed to be done.

'They should be helped and supported to understand that and to do the right thing for their child.

'Very occasionally that might need some statutory intervention but I think it will be very rare.'

She added that the 'vast majority' of child protection investigations and procedures would not result in a child being taken away from their family.

She said: 'Child protection procedures would result in a plan with the family to try to ensure that things are improved and the risks of harm are improved.'

At its annual meeting, the BMA will also debate a series of other measures to tackle obesity. These include calls for a ban on the advertising of junk food; a halt to the sale of school playgrounds and sports fields; and compulsory school exercise of up to an hour a day.

14 June 2007

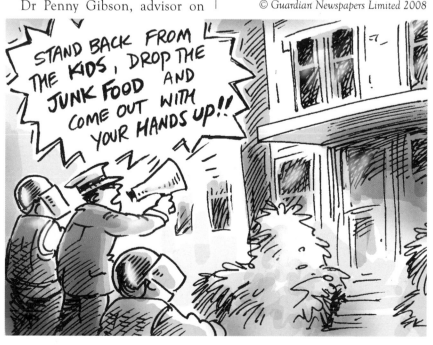

STAND BACK FROM THE KIDS, DROP THE JUNK FOOD AND COME OUT WITH YOUR HANDS UP!!

The answer to childhood obesity

15 minutes of football?

Everyone knows children are getting fatter and that both a poor diet and a lack of exercise are to blame. But, what researchers have been unable to discover until now, is exactly how major a role activity plays in the battle to keep obesity at bay.

Today, a new report published in the journal *PLoS Medicine* offers new hope for parents concerned about the growing obesity epidemic. It suggests that making even small increases to your daily exercise routine, such as walking your child to school each day instead of taking the car, could have dramatic long-term results.

Using the latest cutting-edge techniques, researchers from Bristol University's Children of the 90s project discovered that doing 15 minutes a day of moderate exercise lowered a child's chances of being obese by almost 50 per cent. As long as the activity was at least of the level of a brisk walk – enough to make your child a little out of breath – it seemed to be of benefit.

What makes the results particularly startling is both the large number of UK children studied and the use of high-tech equipment, providing the most accurate measures of both fat and activity levels ever achieved for a study of this type.

Researchers monitored 5,500 12-year-olds from the Children of the 90s research project (also known as ALSPAC, the Avon Longitudinal Study of Parents and Children) based at the University of Bristol, measuring their activity levels for 10 hours a day.

Each child wore a special 'Actigraph activity monitor', which sits on a belt around the waist and records every move they made. Most wore the movement-sensitive monitor for a week but all used the Actigraph for at least three days.

They also had their body fat measured using an X-ray emission scanner, which differentiates both muscle and fat deposits in the body. This is far more precise than the usual BMI (Body Mass Index) system often used to estimate fat levels.

Heading up the research is Professor Chris Riddoch from Bath University together with Children of the 90s' co-director Professor Andy Ness and his team at Bristol.

Doing 15 minutes a day of moderate exercise lowered a child's chances of being obese by almost 50 per cent

---

Professor Riddoch explained the significance of their results, 'This study provides some of the first robust evidence on the link between physical activity and obesity in children.

'We know that diet is important – but what this research tells us is that we mustn't forget about activity. It's been really surprising to us how even small amounts of exercise appear to have dramatic results.'

Professor Ness added, 'The association between physical activity and obesity we observed was strong. These associations suggest that modest increases in physical activity could lead to important reductions in childhood obesity.'

He also stressed that doing 15 minutes of moderate exercise a day should be regarded as a starting point, but one most people would find able to fit into their lifestyle.

The team will now be taking their research further – looking to see if specific patterns of exercise can help achieve even better results.
20 March 2007

⇨ The above information is reprinted with kind permission from the University of Bristol. Visit www.bristol.ac.uk for more information.
© University of Bristol

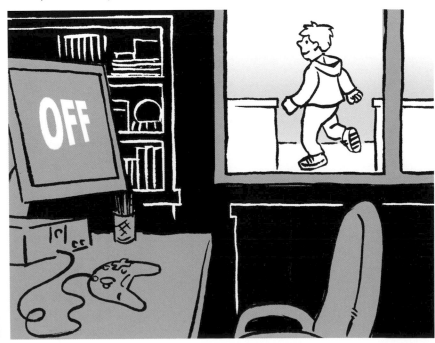

Exercise 'does not make obese children slim'

By Kate Devlin, Medical Correspondent

Encouraging overweight children to exercise has no impact on weight loss and they should be encouraged instead to eat more healthily, according to new research.

The study claims that obese children are inactive because of their weight, and not fat because they are inactive.

The researchers argue that efforts to reduce the childhood obesity epidemic should focus on healthy eating and cutting calorie consumption, rather than getting children to engage in sports and games.

The research, presented at the European Congress on Obesity, studied 300 children over five years.

It found that being overweight influences activity more than activity influences being overweight, and argues that this is why attempts to promote physical activity as a way of combating childhood obesity have failed.

Overweight children find it more difficult to exercise because they run out of breath, so they are more inactive than slimmer counterparts.

The focus of prevention should shift to controlling calorie intake, says the study.

Brad Metcalf, who led the research at the Peninsula Medical School in Plymouth, said: 'Our explanation is that fat kids are inactive because they are fat and not fat because they are inactive. They find it hard to exercise because they run out of breath, and so they don't.

'It is getting them to make sure they do not acquire fats through other means in the first place.

'They will lose more weight through healthy, lifelong changes to their diet than physical activity.

'The most cost-effective way of easing the problem would be to put all the money into getting kids to stop eating junk food rather than splitting it between that and getting them active.

'It is tempting to make kids more active but it doesn't produce the expected results.

'In France, they have taken out vending machines from schools and banned students taking in chocolate bars in their packed lunch. They have also banned adverts for junk food on TV during children's programmes and they are seeing it is making a difference.'

26 May 2008

Physical activity

This article is for people who would like information about the health benefits of physical activity

Keeping physically active can prevent major illnesses such as heart disease, diabetes and colon cancer. Despite this, about two in three men and three in four women do less than 30 minutes' moderate intensity activity on at least five days a week.

Why exercise?

Physical activity can prevent many major illnesses. Evidence shows that regular exercise can:
⇨ promote healthy blood sugar levels to prevent or control diabetes;
⇨ promote bone density to protect against osteoporosis;
⇨ reduce the overall risk of cancer;
⇨ increase levels of HDL or 'good' cholesterol – reducing the risk of developing heart disease;

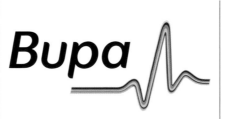

⇨ lower high blood pressure – reducing the risk of developing heart disease;
⇨ boost the immune system;
⇨ boost self-confidence and help prevent depression;
⇨ in combination with a balanced diet, help to maintain a healthy weight.

Barriers to being more active

You may find the threat of a future illness is not enough motivation to change your habits now. There can be many reasons for not taking up exercise, including:
⇨ lack of time due to work or family commitments;
⇨ cost of equipment or gym membership;
⇨ lack of facilities nearby;
⇨ personal safety when exercising outdoors alone;
⇨ poor weather or night-time lighting.

However, there are ways to overcome all of these potential barriers and work exercise into your daily life. This could include getting off the bus to work one or two stops earlier than usual.

What types of activity count?

Many people believe that only vigorous exercise or playing sport counts as healthy activity. Yet substantial health benefits can be achieved from regular activity without the need for special equipment, sporting ability or getting very hot and sweaty.

When you do moderate intensity activity, your breathing and heart rate will increase and you will feel warm. You should still be able to talk without panting in between your words.

Moderate intensity physical activity, such as brisk walking, painting, hoovering and mowing the lawn, all count and are enough to benefit health and prevent illness in adults.

It's possible to achieve your 30 minutes at least five times a week target by making fairly simple changes to your everyday routine – without joining the gym or running a marathon.

Examples of everyday activities that count include:
⇨ walking up stairs instead of using lifts;
⇨ walking up moving escalators;
⇨ walking instead of driving for short journeys;
⇨ doing the housework at double-time;
⇨ DIY and gardening.

How much physical activity should I do?

For an adult weighing 60kg (132lbs), regular, moderate intensity physical activity means using up about an extra 100 calories (kcal) per day, most days of the week. This is about 30 minutes of activity, such as a 1.5 mile (2km) brisk walk.

If you have previously been inactive, separate sessions of 10 or 15 minutes also count and can help you reach the 30-minute amount.

Children and young people need to do 60 minutes of moderate intensity physical activity every day. This needs to include at least two weekly activities that produce high physical stress on bones, such as dancing, jumping or aerobics to aid development.

Getting motivated
Keeping fit

Your ability to keep up a physical activity, such as jogging, racket sports, cycling or swimming, is related to your aerobic fitness or stamina.

Generally speaking, the greater your stamina, the greater are the health benefits. If you want to improve your stamina, it's important to start gently, increasing the frequency of your activity before increasing how hard you exercise.

Have fun

There are many activities you could take part in to increase your stamina. Not everyone sees exercise as fun, and doing something you find boring, just because it's good for you, is very difficult to sustain. But you can take steps to make it more enjoyable.
⇨ Try out different sports or activities until you find something you like, such as a dance or aerobics class.
⇨ Join a team or club where you could meet new friends. This could be a local football team, or a sport you may not have tried before (like korfball).
⇨ Activities that you can do as a family or with friends may help with motivation. When you find an activity you like, exercise at a pace that still allows you to talk.
⇨ Try to go somewhere different and exercise outside such as a forest, a beach or a park.
⇨ Make sure you vary your activity a little so you don't get bored.

Achieving your goals

Even when you usually enjoy exercising, there will be days when you just can't seem to find the motivation to get active. Here are some practical tips to help keep up your enthusiasm.

Substantial health benefits can be achieved from regular activity without the need for special equipment, sporting ability or getting very hot and sweaty

---

⇨ Keep a diary that highlights the sport or activity you do. Note down how far you ran or the match score, your pulse, how you felt, etc. That way you can look back and see how you have improved over time.
⇨ Collect inspiration and stick quotes from coaches, athletes or anyone successful around your house and/or your office. Inspirational stories from people who have achieved against the odds may help – if they can do it, so can you.
⇨ Set yourself some short and long-term goals. Success will provide you with a sense of satisfaction and further motivation to keep up the new lifestyle. Keep your goals: specific; measurable; achievable; realistic; time-based (SMART). For example, rather than saying you'll get fit by summer, start by setting the more specific goal of going to a

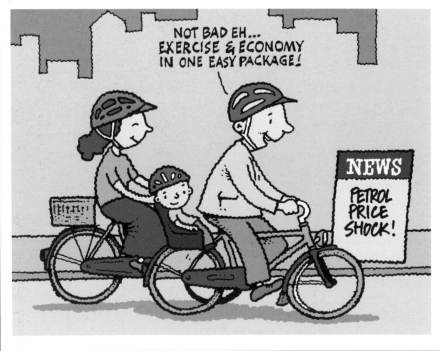

NOT BAD EH... EXERCISE & ECONOMY IN ONE EASY PACKAGE!

NEWS
PETROL PRICE SHOCK!

one-hour step aerobics class or an ashtanga yoga class each week.

Staying motivated

When it comes to staying motivated it's just as important to train your brain as it is to train your body. Here are just a few ideas to help you.

⇨ A great way to stay focused is to keep reminding yourself of the reasons you started exercising in the first place. This may include losing excess weight, improving your health or testing yourself in a competition or race.

> When it comes to staying motivated it's just as important to train your brain as it is to train your body

⇨ Picture yourself achieving your goal, such as completing a race or fitting into smaller trousers – and imagine what it will feel like. Through visualisation these images and feelings will motivate you and will help you achieve them for real.

⇨ Exercising releases chemicals in the brain, like serotonin, that have a strong effect on your mood, helping reduce anxiety, stress and depression. So whenever you don't feel like exercising, try to remind yourself how good you'll feel afterwards.

Further information

⇨ British Heart Foundation National Centre for Physical Activity and Health (HFNC)
www.bhfactive.org.uk

Sources

⇨ Bone health for all. National Osteoporosis Society
www.nos.org.uk
accessed 18 January 2007
⇨ Evidence on the impact of physical activity and its relationship to health. A report from the Chief Medical Officer. Department of Health, At least five a week: April 2004.
www.dh.gov.uk
⇨ Exercise and depression. Mental

Health Foundation
www.mentalhealth.org.uk
accessed 18 January 2007
⇨ Physical activity and your heart. Heart Information Series Number 1 booklet. The British Heart Foundation. July 2005
www.bhf.org.uk
⇨ Why is it important to you? Diabetes UK
www.diabetes.org.uk
accessed 1 November 2006

This information was published by BUPA's health information team and is based on reputable sources of medical evidence. It has been peer reviewed by Dr James Quekett, Bsc. MB Ch.B MRCGP DRCOG DFFP, partner/principal general practitioner at Rowcroft Medical Centre, and by BUPA doctors. The content is intended for general information only and does not replace the need for personal advice from a qualified health professional.
August 2007

⇨ The above information is re-printed with kind permission from Bupa. Visit www.bupa.co.uk for more.
© Bupa

Reasons not to exercise

Written by Anne-Marie Millard, personal fitness instructor

We are surrounded by advice that says we need to keep fit, keep our hearts healthy and our cholesterol count low – so much so, we sometimes overlook the fact there are times when we shouldn't be exercising at all.

1. When you're ill

Don't exercise when you're unwell, even if it is just a cold.

Exercise will put more strain on your immune system and prolong illness. This will result in you spending more time away from your fitness programme.

It's also a prime cause of other injuries because it is more difficult to concentrate on what you're doing if you're feeling ill.

I've seen someone faint while doing a step class with a high temperature, and get a black eye from hitting her neighbour's step.

2. When you haven't had enough recuperation time

Don't rush back to your normal exercise routine after you have been ill. Starting to exercise too early is

It is not advisable to exercise whilst ill

likely to lead to a re-emergence of your symptoms.

When you do decide to return to the gym, make sure you start your workout slowly and with care.

Even a week or so off your usual routine can make a difference. Ease yourself back into your programme by doing just 50 per cent of your normal workload and gradually building up.

3. When you're feeling wiped out and stressed

There will be days when you don't feel like going to the gym, but sometimes your body can be telling you to take a break.

It can do you a power of good to have a day off from your fitness programme.

Go home, have a healthy meal: don't mentally punish yourself for not going to the gym.

Remember: all-round fitness incorporates spiritual wellbeing. Even though exercise can give us that stress-lifting endorphin high, sometimes we just need to relax.

4. When you have an injury

Whatever your injury, make sure that it is thoroughly healed before you go back to training.

A simple injury can be made much worse by your well-meaning attempt to 'loosen it up'. You could injure yourself again, but worse.

Seek professional advice from a physiotherapist or osteopath for any strain or sports injury that is still painful after 24 hours.

5. When you haven't got the correct equipment

Whatever your sport is, make sure you buy the best equipment you can afford. Don't just follow the fad for the latest trendy trainers or gear.

Not having the right equipment can result in injury.

Take footwear seriously. A good sports shop will have well-trained staff who can properly assist you in choosing the correct shoes for your needs. For example, there are different types of trainers for running, depending on your natural step.

⇨ Normal foot: will leave a wet footprint that has a curve on one side, but shows the top part of the foot and heel connected by a broad band. A normal foot lands on the outside of the heel and rolls inwards slightly to absorb shock. This means you are running efficiently and don't need a motion control shoe.

⇨ Flat foot: has a low arch and leaves a footprint that looks like the whole sole of the foot. When running, the foot strikes the outside of the heel and rolls inwards (pronates) too much, which can cause injury. Motion control or stability shoes can help.

⇨ High-arched foot: will leave a footprint that has a highly curved band between the top part of the foot and heel. In some cases there is no band at all. When running, the heel doesn't roll inwards enough to absorb shock. Cushioned shoes with lots of flexibility can help.

Other forms of exercise equipment such as horse-riding gear should be bought from a professional supplier.

6. When you've got a hangover

If you've got a hangover from the night before, think twice before going to your morning aerobics class.

All-round fitness incorporates spiritual wellbeing. Even though exercise can give us that stress-lifting endorphin high, sometimes we just need to relax

---

Alcohol dehydrates you, so make sure you have drunk enough water to balance out its effects.

Ask yourself if you are still under the influence: it takes the body about an hour to process one unit of alcohol. If you have had four pints of beer, it won't be out of your system for eleven hours.

Don't exercise if there is any chance that you are still drunk.

Think about when you last ate. Sometimes eating breakfast with a hangover is the last thing you want to do, but if you haven't taken in enough fuel to train, don't do it.

7. When you're pregnant

The rules about exercising in pregnancy form a whole book in themselves, so we're just going to touch on the subject.

The main points are that you can exercise throughout your pregnancy as long as a) you feel like it and b) your GP and midwife have said you can.

While the advice is to keep fit throughout your pregnancy, the emphasis is on maintaining fitness, not improving. Pregnancy is a nine-month workout in itself.

If you decide to exercise when pregnant, get professional advice after your third month on what you should and should not do.

8. After your baby is born

How many celebrities do we hear boasting that they went straight back to 300 sit-ups per day within 24 hours of childbirth?

Firstly, I wouldn't believe a word of it, and secondly they would be going against all health guidelines if they did.

However desperate you are to retrieve your figure, you have to wait six weeks before you can start gently exercising, or 12 weeks if you've had a C-section.

After this time, start slowly, gradually building up to your pre-pregnancy exercise routine. And get professional advice about which sort of abdominal exercises you should be doing post-baby.

An area that causes a lot of silent embarrassment is the pelvic floor muscle. If you have done work on it during pregnancy you shouldn't have too much trouble, but get some specific exercises set down for you to help prevent leakage.

What if I just lack motivation?

The main piece of advice is to be sensible: think about your motives for exercising and why you don't want to exercise.

Be honest with yourself. If you really just can't be bothered, maybe you are finding your exercise programme boring.

If that's the case, it's time you shook up your routine a little. Try adding new forms of exercise that interest you such as in-line skating, dance classes or aqua aerobics.

Finally, remember how many times you've said: 'I don't feel like it' and come away saying: 'I'm really glad I did that!'
25 July 2007

⇨ The above information is re-printed with kind permission from NetDoctor. Visit www.netdoctor.co.uk for more information.

© *NetDoctor*

The fitness myths

If you believe running is bad for the knees or that yoga helps a sore back, then think again, writes Peta Bee

Working out can be not only tough and time-consuming, it is often downright bamboozling. Listen to all the advice about which sort of exercise to choose and you might be excused for wanting to hang up your trainers in despair. Wouldn't it help simplify gym matters if we looked at how the five biggest fitness myths stack up against scientific fact?

> **Scientific studies cast considerable doubt on the possibility of selectively taking inches off the waist, thighs or buttocks**

Myth: You can spot-reduce fat from any part of the body

The diet and fitness industries have traded for so long on the concept of targeting specific body parts for fat removal – hip-and-thigh eating plans, bums, tums and thighs workouts etc. – that quite a few people have actually come to believe that spot-reduction is possible. But scientific studies cast considerable doubt on the possibility of selectively taking inches off the waist, thighs or buttocks. Dr Cedric Bryant, chief science officer for the American Council on Exercise, a consumer watchdog for the fitness industry, says there is little evidence to support such claims. One landmark study designed to test the spot-reduction theory was carried out at the University of Massachusetts where 13 male subjects did a vigorous abdominal exercise programme for one month. Each subject performed a total of 5,000 sit-ups over 27 days. But when fat biopsies from their stomachs, buttocks and upper backs obtained at the beginning and end of

the trial were analysed, fat loss proved similar at all three sites, not just the abdomen. 'If caloric expenditure is enough, it will cause fat from the entire body, including that from a target area, to be reduced,' Bryant says. 'However, although fat is lost from the entire body through exercise and calorie reduction, it appears that the last areas to become lean tend to be those areas where an individual tends to gain fat first. For most men, that is the abdominal region and for women it is hips, buttocks and thighs.'

Myth: Running is bad for your knees

Slapping the pavement with the soles of your trainers has gained running a reputation as public enemy number one to the knee joint. But a recent study showed instead that running actually protects those joints from damage and pain. Reporting in the journal *Arthritis Research and Therapy*, a team from the department of immunology and rheumatology at Stanford University in southern California found that adults who run consistently can expect to have 25% less musculoskeletal pain and less arthritis than non-runners when they get older.

Dr Bonnie Bruce, the study author, followed more than 500 runners from

a local club (called 'ever runners' in the study) and 300 inactive people ('never runners', but not necessarily sedentary) in their 50s and 60s for 14 years. When results from an annual health questionnaire were analysed, Bruce and her colleagues found that the 'ever runners', who ran at least six hours per week on average, experienced less joint pain by their 60s and 70s and only 35% of the joggers got arthritis (compared to 43% of non-runners).

Sammy Margo, a sports physiotherapist for the Chartered Society of Physiotherapy, says running doesn't deserve its bad press. 'The key is consistency,' Margo says. 'If you run consistently, your joints, tendons, ligaments, disks and muscles get used to the habitual pounding of the activity. The body accommodates and copes with the demands.'

It is the yo-yo runners, says Margo, who take up jogging and then drop it repeatedly over a number of years who might have problems after a while.

Myth: Yoga is good for back pain

Contorting yourself like a pretzel on a yoga mat may be good for many things but not, apparently, for your back. In a study published in the *Annals of Internal Medicine*, researchers

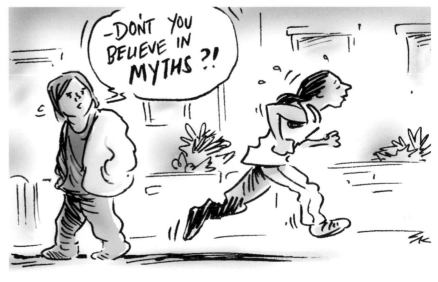

found that a gentle yoga class seemed a better alternative to 'either general exercise or a self-help book' for back pain. However, Dr Karen Sherman who conducted the study conceded that more vigorous types of yoga, such as ashtanga, and classes led by poorly qualified instructors, can potentially make problems worse. Matt Todman, consultant physiotherapist at the Sports and Spinal Clinic, Harley Street, goes further, saying: 'yoga is generally not good for back pain and a lot of its postures can compound the problem by loading pressure on the back'.

Widely regarded as the core targets of exercising: three to five times a week for 20 to 60 minutes at 55-90% of your body's maximum capacity

---

Staying active, though, is important, although back-pain sufferers should do so only on the advice of their physiotherapist. Jeremy Fairbank, consultant orthopaedic surgeon at the Nuffield Hospital, Oxford, found that patients obtain as much benefit from an intense programme of exercise therapy as from spinal surgery. Fairbank's trial, funded by the Medical Research Council and involving almost 350 patients, revealed that those who followed a tailored daily exercise programme involving activities such as step-ups, walking on a treadmill, cycling and core stability work for five days over three weeks made huge progress.

Myth: Pilates will give you a celebrity body

Fans are reported to include Madonna, Jodie Foster and Liz Hurley, but while the cult gym practice might leave you with a super-strong core or middle-section, it will do little to improve your cardiovascular fitness and lower body fat, at least according to the results of a study last year by the American Council on Exercise (ACE). Professor John Pocari and his team of exercise scientists at the University of Wisconsin analysed the demands of 50-minute beginner and advanced level Pilates classes and found the intensity of each to be lower than the recommended level for improving cardiovascular fitness.

In the beginners' classes, the maximum heart rate of the healthy and moderately fit female subjects was only 54% when the accepted range for boosting fitness is 64-94%. They burned 175 calories. Even the advanced class failed to raise heart rates above an average 62% and burned only 254 calories, equivalent to the benefits gained from walking at a slow pace. In order to get fitter and slimmer, the experts suggested that Pilates is done in conjunction with aerobic activities such as running or cycling. 'Pilates has a long list of benefits including improved body mechanics, balance, coordination, strength and flexibility,' says Dr Cedric Bryant of ACE. 'A Pilates session burns a relatively small amount of calories, but it is still a valuable addition to an exercise routine.'

Myth: You don't need to 'feel the burn' to get fitter

Current government recommendations suggest that totting up half an hour of activity by performing tasks such as housework, gardening or collecting the newspaper is enough to ward off heart disease and keep us healthy.

But these are minimum requirements (even though two-thirds of men and three-quarters of women barely manage to meet them) and if you really want to shape up, it requires a lot more sweat and toil.

Research by the American College of Sports Medicine (ACSM) sets what are widely regarded as the core targets of exercising three to five times a week for 20 to 60 minutes at 55-90% of your body's maximum capacity, calculated according to your heart rate, if you want to improve fitness. 'That constitutes a fairly vigorous workout that would leave you breathless and puffing,' says Dr Greg Whyte, sports science coordinator for the English Institute of Sport. 'And it is the level you need to be doing if you want to get fitter.'

That doesn't mean we can rest on our laurels for the rest of the time. Whyte believes too many people have 'reached a point where they think going to the gym three times a week is enough'. But, he says, while working out will contribute considerably towards overall fitness, 'there are 23 and a bit hours remaining in the day and we should try to be active at least during some of them'.

It doesn't end there. Louise Sutton, senior lecturer in health and exercise science at Leeds Metropolitan University, says that there has to be an element of progression in a workout regimen. 'The body and its muscles respond to the overload principle,' she says. 'And there comes a time when you will need to extend the duration or intensity of your exercise to get fitter still.'

5 June 2007

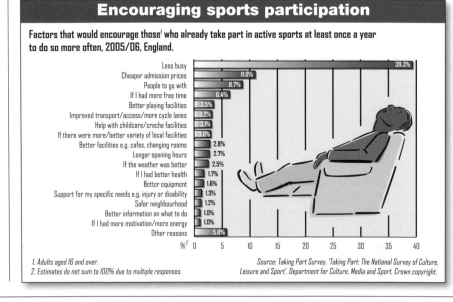

Encouraging sports participation

Factors that would encourage those[1] who already take part in active sports at least once a year to do so more often, 2005/06, England.

Factor	%
Less busy	39.3%
Cheaper admission prices	11.0%
People to go with	8.7%
If I had more free time	6.4%
Better playing facilities	3.5%
Improved transport/access/more cycle lanes	3.2%
Help with childcare/creche facilities	3.1%
If there were more/better variety of local facilities	3.0%
Better facilities e.g. cafes, changing rooms	2.8%
Longer opening hours	2.7%
If the weather was better	2.5%
If I had better health	1.7%
Better equipment	1.6%
Support for my specific needs e.g. injury or disability	1.3%
Safer neighbourhood	1.2%
Better information on what to do	1.0%
If I had more motivation/more energy	1.0%
Other reasons	5.8%

%[2] 0 5 10 15 20 25 30 35 40

1. Adults aged 16 and over.
2. Estimates do not sum to 100% due to multiple responses.

Source: Taking Part Survey. 'Taking Part: The National Survey of Culture, Leisure and Sport'. Department for Culture, Media and Sport. Crown copyright.

Keep-fit boom fails to stem obesity

The booming fitness industry has done little to curb the obesity epidemic, according to leading academic researchers

While gyms and private health clubs have grown in popularity in recent years, the nation's weight has grown too.

The reason for the paradox, they said, is that such clubs tend to attract wealthier people, leaving the less well-off struggling to find ways to combat weight problems.

Gyms, fitness magazines and manuals often focus on keeping in shape for image reasons rather than for health reasons, claimed the University of Leicester study.

The industry has been able to make a profit by attracting richer members using 'seductive marketing' without providing a 'sustainable approach to fitness', it concluded.

The findings, compiled by Dr Jennifer Smith Maguire of the university's department of media and communications, focused on the US, which has more than 20,000 commercial health clubs.

But the rapid growth in private clubs in the UK means the research can be applied here, she said.

'Over recent decades, many Western countries have experienced a strange paradox, with fitness and exercise industries expanding alongside problems of inactivity and obesity,' said Dr Smith Maguire.

'The commercial fitness industry benefits from the scientific legitimacy and political urgency bestowed on population health issues, such as inactivity and obesity.

While gyms and private health clubs have grown in popularity in recent years, the nation's weight has grown too

---

'But it is ill-equipped to address those issues for a number of reasons.'

She added: 'In the US, for example, half of commercial health club members are in the top 20 per cent of income earners.

'At the top end of the market, high income earners can afford excellent services and an enlightened approach to fitness, but at the bottom end of the market, middle and lower income earners can afford fewer and lower quality services and a factory approach to fitness.

'And at the very bottom, excluded altogether from the market, are those individuals most likely to be inactive and obese.'

Dr Smith Maguire said: 'The fitness industry perpetuates the idea that health is an individual matter.'

But she argued that inactivity and obesity are problems for society as a whole and they require collective solutions.

'Physical exercise can be re-introduced as an integral part of everyday life, rather than yet another activity to be squeezed into an already shrinking supply of free time.'

A Government report warned last month that one in two women and 60 per cent of men will be obese by 2050. Obesity is projected to cost the country £45billion a year by 2050.

By then, only 10 per cent of men and 15 per cent of women will be the right weight for their height.

6 November 2007

⇨ The above information is reprinted with kind permission from This is London. Visit www.thisislondon.co.uk for more information.

© *This is London*

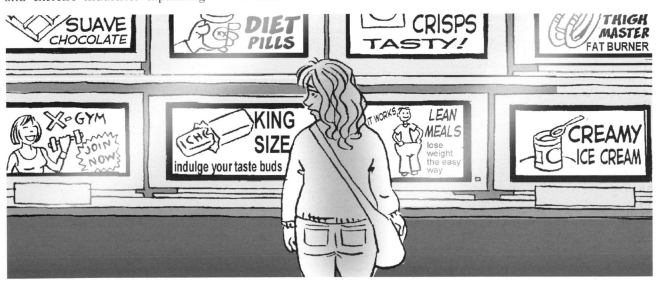

Study tips the scales in favour of exercise

Information from the University of Leeds

People who are overweight or obese shouldn't give up exercise even if they fail to lose much weight, according to a new study from the University of Leeds, which found the health benefits of exercise go well beyond dropping a dress size.

As part of the study, 58 overweight men and women completed a 12-week cardio-exercise regime, involving five supervised training sessions a week, designed to burn 500 calories each time.

By the end, some individuals had lost up to 14.7kg in weight, the average weight loss was 3.7kg, while others lost less weight than expected. But most surprisingly, five people had actually gained 1-2kg. Clearly then, regular exercise doesn't have the same effects on everyone.

However, Professor John Blundell from the Leeds BioPsychology Group said what is more significant is that all of the participants reaped the benefits of a drop in blood pressure, reduced body fat, a smaller waist, and a slower heart rate.

'The results showed that although there were great variations in weight loss between individuals, you still get a lot of extra benefits from doing exercise that you wouldn't get from dieting alone, even if you don't lose any pounds,' he said.

Dr Neil King, the co-principal investigator, added: 'Everyone who took part in this study was able to exercise at a higher intensity level, so they all got fitter. For example, their maximum oxygen consumption, called VO2 max, increased by an average of 20% after just 12 weeks. So on balance, it's probably better to be fit and overweight, rather than slim but unfit.'

Most astonishingly, even in the group of people who lost little or no weight, their blood pressure dropped significantly, and they typically lost 3.7cm off their waist circumference, which is equivalent to one dress or trouser size.

'Waist circumference indicates how much fat you carry in your abdomen area, which is a strong risk factor for heart disease in men and women,' he explained. They also burned off between 1.5% and 3.5% fat mass and gained lean tissue, so their body composition was visibly changing.

The health benefits of exercise go well beyond dropping a dress size

The findings of the BBSRC-funded study were published last month in the *International Journal of Obesity*. The other Leeds researchers involved were Mark Hopkins and Phillipa Caudwell, together with academics from the Queensland University of Technology in Brisbane.

This is the first time that a major exercise study has monitored people during training sessions to ensure they all did exactly the same workout. Often exercise fails to produce a desired weight loss because of lack of compliance.

Professor Blundell said the results suggest that biological differences may partly be to blame for obesity, as in some individuals physical activity can trigger a compensatory response and try to 'steal back calories' after exercise. For example, their body might respond to the energy deficit by stimulating their appetite, causing them to snack more on energy dense high-fat foods, being more inactive at other times of the day, or by slowing their metabolic rate.

'People often overestimate how much energy they have burned off through exercise,' he said. 'To shed 600 kilocalories, for example, a moderately fit person would have to exercise for about 60 minutes. Yet it only takes three minutes to eat 600 kilocalories in the form of a piece of gateau and a Danish pastry.'

The study also asked participants to wear heart rate monitors and activity meters every day to calculate how much energy they used at other times. The initial results suggest some people may involuntarily rest more before or after exercise to compensate for the energy deficit.

'We strongly advocate the role of exercise in weight management, however, its effectiveness will vary between individuals.

'Our results suggest that the body's response to exercise can act as a major barrier to weight loss, so some people probably won't lose weight through exercise alone, and may need extra help to keep their appetite in check,' said Professor Blundell.

The challenge now for science is to figure out why exercise helps some people lose weight but not others. The research team have collected a large number of blood samples to look for the presence of certain peptides known to influence human appetite, and they suspect that physical activity may drive up these peptides.

'We're also following up with the 58 people who did this study to find out if they've reverted to their original body weight or lost more weight. We're starting the exercise sessions up again in January with a new group of volunteers and will be looking in greater detail at those who don't lose any weight.'
29 October 2007

⇨ The above information is reprinted with kind permission from the University of Leeds. Visit www.leeds.ac.uk for more information.
© University of Leeds

Boost mental health

Fitness doesn't just help with physical health, it can have a positive effect on your mind, and is especially helpful in treating mild depression

⇨ A survey carried out by the charity Mind in 2001 found that 83% of people with mental health problems looked to exercise to help lift their mood or to reduce stress. Two-thirds said exercise helped to relieve the symptoms of depression and more than half said it helped to reduce stress and anxiety. Six out of 10 of the respondents said that physical exercise helped to improve their motivation, 50% said it boosted their self-esteem and 24% said it improved their social skills.

83% of people with mental health problems looked to exercise to help lift their mood or to reduce stress

---

⇨ Exercise gives you a natural high. This is because it causes the brain to release serotonin, dopamine, norepinephrine, and endorphins which are known to have strong effects on mood, helping to reduce feelings of anxiety, stress and mild to moderate depression. One of the main benefits of using exercise to help lift depression is that you start to feel effects instantly, unlike drugs which can take several weeks to kick in.

⇨ Researchers at Duke University, Carolina, USA, studied people suffering from depression for four months and found that 60% of the participants who exercised for 30 minutes three times a week overcame their depression without using antidepressant medication. This is the same percentage rate as for those who only used medication in their treatment for depression.

⇨ Being more active aids sleep, and as sleep problems are commonly associated with depression it can help with this condition.

⇨ By feeling (and gradually looking) fitter and healthier, exercise allows people to gain a more positive body image, as well as boosting their self-confidence and self-esteem. This in turn means that they can begin to socialise with more ease.

⇨ Regular exercise also reduces stress and tension, and helps clear the mind. It enables people to unwind and relax in the evenings rather than dwell on problems.

⇨ It boosts energy levels, something those with depression commonly lack. Once you've forced yourself to go and do some exercise the first few times you'll soon find yourself feeling more energetic, even if you just go for short walks.

⇨ The above information is reprinted with kind permission from TheSite. Visit www.thesite.org for more information.

© TheSite

Obesity risk for 'moderately active' Britons

Information from Private Healthcare UK

Health guidelines issued by the government need to be modified to ensure the health and fitness levels of Britons are improved, it has been claimed.

Research conducted by scientists at the University of Exeter and Brunel University suggests that current rules need to be reassessed in order to reduce the burden of obesity, type two diabetes and heart disease on society.

At present, the Department of Health recommends that Britons partake in 30 minutes of moderate exercise – which can include activities such as walking, housework or gardening – a total of five times a week in order to remain healthy.

As a result, 56 per cent of men and 71 per cent of women are now of the belief that walking a few times a week is enough for them to keep in good shape and steer clear of health problems.

However, the researchers found that 'maximal protection from disease' is only attainable through vigorous exercise such as jogging and running.

'Time and time again, the largest and most robust studies have shown that vigorously active individuals live longer and enjoy a better quality of life than moderately active individuals and couch potatoes,' the study's lead author, Dr Gary O'Donovan, commented.

'It's extremely worrying that British adults now believe that a brief stroll and a bit of gardening is enough to make them fit and healthy.

'The challenge now is to amend Britain's physical activity guidelines so that they emphasise the role vigorous activity plays in fighting obesity, type two diabetes, and heart disease,' he concluded.

11 October 2007

⇨ The above information is reprinted with kind permission from Private Healthcare UK. Visit www.privatehealth.co.uk for more information.

© Adfero Ltd

Exercise on par with drugs for aiding depression

By Amy Norton

Regular exercise may work as well as medication in improving symptoms of major depression, researchers have found.

In a study of 202 depressed adults, investigators found that those who went through group-based exercise therapy did as well as those treated with an antidepressant drug. A third group that performed home-based exercise also improved, though to a lesser degree.

Importantly, the researchers found, all three groups did better than a fourth group given a placebo – an inactive pill identical to the antidepressant.

While past studies have suggested that exercise can ease depression symptoms, a criticism has been that the research failed to compare exercise with a placebo. This leaves a question as to whether the therapy, per se, was responsible for the benefit.

The new findings bolster evidence that exercise does have a real effect on depression, according to the researchers.

Doctors may not start widely prescribing exercise as a depression treatment just yet. But for patients who are motivated to try exercise, it could be a reasonable option, the study authors say.

'If exercise were a drug, I'm not sure that it would receive FDA approval at this time,' noted study author Dr James A. Blumenthal, a professor of medical psychology at Duke University Medical Center in Durham, North Carolina.

'But,' he told Reuters Health, 'there is certainly growing evidence that exercise may be a viable alternative to medication, at least among those patients who are receptive to exercise as a potential treatment for their depression.'

The study, published in the journal *Psychosomatic Medicine*, included 202 men and women age 40 and older who were diagnosed with major depression. They were randomly assigned to one of four groups: one that worked out in a supervised, group setting three times per week; one that exercised at home; one that took the antidepressant sertraline (Zoloft); and one that took placebo pills.

After 16 weeks, the patients completed standard measures of depression symptoms.

By the end of the study, Blumenthal's team found, 47 per cent of patients on the antidepressant no longer met the criteria for major depression. The same was true of 45 per cent of those in the supervised exercise group.

In the home-based exercise group, 40 per cent had their symptoms go into remission. That compared with 31 per cent of the placebo group.

There are several theories on why exercise might improve depression. For example, physical activity seems to affect some key nervous system chemicals – norepinephrine and serotonin – that are targets of antidepressant drugs, as well as brain neurotrophins, which help protect nerve cells from injury and transmit signals in brain regions related to mood.

Exercise may also boost people's feelings of self-efficacy and promote positive thinking. Some experts speculate that group exercise, with its social aspect, may have added benefits.

Though the home exercise group in this study did better than the placebo group, it's not clear whether it's as good as supervised classes, according to Blumenthal. 'Home exercise may be more convenient,' he noted, 'but patients do not push themselves as hard on their own.'

Regular exercise may work as well as medication in improving symptoms of major depression

He added that supervised exercise may also be safer for some people, such as those with heart disease.

SOURCE: *Psychosomatic Medicine, September 2007*

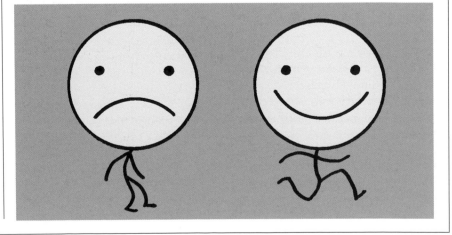

Compulsive exercise

Compulsive exercise is also known as obligatory exercise, excessive exercise, exercise addiction and anorexia athletica, and it describes a compulsion to exercise for longer and more vigorously than what is considered 'normal'

Compulsive exercise does not necessarily always occur alongside an eating disorder, but it is often one of the first signs that someone may be developing a negative relationship with food and possibly an eating disorder such as anorexia.

Exercise is a good thing if it's done for the right reasons, that is, to improve or maintain physical fitness and overall general health.

But exercising at very vigorous levels and for prolonged periods of time can be bad for health, even dangerous.

Too much exercise

Someone who becomes addicted to exercise may start off with normal, good intentions to be fit and healthy, but the number and intensity of exercise sessions gradually increases until they develop a dependency on exercising. As things get out of control, exercise becomes not so much a choice any more as a need.

How much exercise is too much? This is a grey area. Doing more than the government recommended amount (at least 30 minutes of moderate intensity physical activity, on five days of the week) does not automatically mean someone is doing too much.

Signs of compulsive exercise

Here are the signs that someone may have an unhealthy compulsion to exercise:

A compulsive exerciser exercises at length (perhaps for one to two hours or more), most days or every day, sometimes several times each day, often at a vigorous intensity, including when they are feeling unwell or have an injury. Exercise is not undertaken as a fun or pleasurable experience.

Exercising in unusual places and at odd times is not uncommon, such as in bed, in the middle of the night, even in the shower, as the person becomes secretive about their behaviour and tries to hide the amount of exercise they are doing.

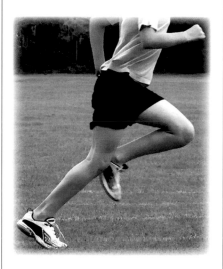

Exercising at very vigorous levels and for prolonged periods of time can be bad for health, even dangerous

Exercise interferes with normal everyday life, taking priority over everything, with all other activities planned around it. This is likely to result in the person becoming withdrawn, and not doing things such as socialising with friends and spending time with family.

The person feels guilty and anxious if they are forced to miss an exercise session, perhaps due to illness, injury or other commitments. If a session is missed, they may try to make up for it at the next one by exercising harder and for longer, or by not eating. Sitting still may sometimes be difficult because it feels like a missed opportunity to do more exercise.

People who exercise excessively often suffer from anxiety and depression, poor body image perception and low self-esteem, and worry about their weight (as is often the case in people with eating disorders). Exercise becomes a way of dealing with these emotions and gaining a sense of control over their lives, while their sense of self-worth is often based on the number and intensity of exercise sessions they can fit in.

Serious health effects of compulsive exercise

There is a real risk of injury and permanent damage to bones, muscles, joints, ligaments and tendons due to the excessive demands placed on the body, especially if it is not allowed to rest and heal.

In addition to this, if adequate nutrients are not consumed, muscles literally begin to waste away, as the body resorts to breaking down muscle mass as a source of energy.

For women, excessive exercise affects the balance of hormones, leading to amenorrhea (absence of the menstrual cycle), fertility problems and osteoporosis (bone loss). It also makes people more susceptible to infections, fatigue and exhaustion as the body is pushed beyond its limits. Unnecessary stress is placed on the heart.

Compulsive exercise and eating disorders

In the context of an eating disorder, compulsive exercise can be considered a form of purging, whereby an attempt is made to get rid of calories and prevent or reverse the effects of putting food into the body. The amount and type of exercise undertaken will be decided after a careful calculation of how much food has been eaten and how many calories need to be burned.

Eating very little and exercising too much is a dangerous combination, and can be very serious, even fatal.

⇨ The above information is reprinted with kind permission from Disordered Eating. Visit www.disordered-eating.co.uk for more information.

© Disordered Eating

KEY FACTS

⇨ The Department of Health predicts that if current trends continues, by 2010 around 6.6 million men will be obese compared to 6 million women. (page 1)

⇨ A minority medical condition 50 years ago, the prevalence of obesity is now such that it is regarded as a major public health issue and listed as a priority by senior government ministers. (page 4)

⇨ By 2050, obesity is expected to increase to 60 per cent of men and 50 per cent of women. (page 5)

⇨ In 2006, 16% of children aged 2 to 15 were classed as obese. This represents an overall increase from 11% in 1995. Despite the overall increase since 1995, the proportion of girls aged 2 to 15 who were obese decreased between 2005 and 2006, from 18% to 15%. There was no significant decrease among boys aged 2 to 15 over that period. Among children aged 2 to 10, 15% were classed as obese in 2006. (page 6)

⇨ Worldwide, 400 million adults are obese and 1.6 billion are overweight. (page 7)

⇨ Worldwide, 155 million children are overweight, including 30-45 million obese children. (page 7)

⇨ Of all the factors that contribute to obesity, hormonal and glandular defects are thought to be the least important, being demonstrable in only about 5% of all obese individuals. (page 8)

⇨ A section of genetic code that puts half the population at greater risk of obesity, diabetes and heart disease has been discovered by scientists who say those carrying the sequence are on average 2kg (4.4lb) heavier than others, with 2cm larger waistlines and a tendency to become resistant to insulin and vulnerable to late-onset diabetes. (page 9)

⇨ The technological revolution of the 20th century has led to weight gain becoming inevitable for most people, because our bodies and biological make-up are out of step with our surroundings, says the latest report from Foresight. (page 10)

⇨ Every 15 minutes someone dies as a direct result of physical inactivity. Yet just 30 minutes of activity a day will help stave off heart disease and other illnesses, according to the British Heart Foundation. (page 11)

⇨ People who do plenty of exercise appear to be biologically younger than those who lead a sedentary lifestyle, researchers have found. (page 12)

⇨ According to the World Health Organisation, 20 per cent of children across Europe are overweight. (page 13)

⇨ The world's largest chronic health problem is not HIV/AIDS but obesity. (page 13)

⇨ Less than three per cent of UK 11-year-olds are taking enough exercise, suggests research. (page 15)

⇨ The NHS costs attributable to overweight and obesity are projected to double to £10 billion per year by 2050. The wider costs to society and business are estimated to reach £49.9 billion per year (at today's prices). (page 19)

⇨ A review of research examining the effectiveness of different obesity treatments has concluded that no matter what other forms of therapy are offered, changes in lifestyle are imperative if patients want to maximise and maintain their weight loss. (page 20)

⇨ Obesity costs the economy up to £3.7bn and accounts for 18 million sick days per year. (page 21)

⇨ 68% of employers believe obesity is a serious issue in the workplace, contributing to lower productivity and higher costs. (page 21)

⇨ Researchers from Bristol University's Children of the 90s project discovered that doing 15 minutes a day of moderate exercise lowered a child's chances of being obese by almost 50 per cent. As long as the activity was at least of the level of a brisk walk – enough to make a child a little out of breath – it seemed to be of benefit. (page 28)

⇨ Encouraging overweight children to exercise has no impact on weight loss and they should be encouraged instead to eat more healthily, according to research from the Peninsula Medical School in Plymouth. (page 29)

⇨ For an adult weighing 60kg (132lbs), regular, moderate intensity physical activity means using up about an extra 100 calories (kcal) per day, most days of the week. This is about 30 minutes of activity, such as a 1.5 mile (2km) brisk walk. (page 30)

⇨ 39.3% of people surveyed who already took part in active sports at least once a year claimed they would do so more often if they were less busy. (page 34)

⇨ People who are overweight or obese shouldn't give up exercise even if they fail to lose much weight, according to a new study from the University of Leeds, which found the health benefits of exercise go well beyond dropping a dress size. (page 36)

GLOSSARY

Blood pressure
A measure of the force of the blood on the artery walls when the heart beats. High blood pressure increases the risk of developing cardiovascular disease and circulatory illnesses.

Body Mass Index (BMI)
A measurement that compares an individual's weight against their height to determine if they are within healthy weight guidelines. BMI is calculated by taking a person's weight in kilogrammes and dividing it by the square of their height in metres. A BMI between 18.5 and 25 is considered 'normal' – that is, a healthy weight for your height.

Calorie
A unit used to measure the amount of energy the body gets from food. Confusingly, what we tend to refer to in everyday speech as a 'calorie' is in reality a kilocalorie (abbreviated 'kcal' on food labelling). Your body needs a certain amount of calories each day, but eating more than the recommended daily amount causes excess energy to be stored as fat. The recommended daily allowance (RDA) of calories is 2000 for women and 2,500 for men.

Compulsive exercise
This occurs when a person feels psychologically compelled to exercise more than would generally be considered 'normal', sometimes to the detriment of their health, and feels guilty or anxious when they can't exercise. It may precede or accompany an eating disorder, but this is not always the case.

Cardiovascular disease (CVD)
Refers to diseases of the heart or blood vessels. The main causes of cardiovascular disease are smoking, physical inactivity, poor diet and being overweight. Cardiovascular disease is the most common cause of death in the UK.

Coronary disease
Occurs when the arteries that carry blood and oxygen to the heart are narrowed by a build-up of fatty material in their walls, which can lead to angina or a heart attack.

Cholesterol
A type of fat produced by the body. Although cholesterol is needed for the body to function normally, a high cholesterol level puts you at risk of heart disease and stroke.

Diabetes
A chronic disease in which there is too much sugar in the blood. This occurs because the body does not produce enough insulin, or because it cannot use it properly. Type 2, or adult-onset, diabetes has been linked to rising rates of obesity.

Exercise
Physical activity undertaken in order to maintain fitness and health.

'Fattism'
A term used to describe discrimination against overweight people.

Obesity
Obesity is a condition which occurs when, due to the accumulation of excess body fat, an individual becomes severely overweight and their BMI exceeds 30. Obesity can cause serious health problems and increases the risk of developing diseases such as heart disease, diabetes and some types of cancer. Obesity is a growing problem, caused mainly by poor diet and a lack of physical activity. Worldwide, 400 million adults and 30-45 million children are obese.

Overweight
A person is considered overweight if their BMI is between 25 and 30. According to government statistics, one in four men and one in three women in the UK are overweight.

Physical activity
Physical activity is any movement which increases the amount of energy expended by the muscles. Physical activity can lower the risk of developing many illnesses and it is recommended that adults should take at least 30 minutes of moderate physical activity on at least five days during the week.

Weight loss surgery
Also known as bariatric surgery, this type of medical procedure is only available to those considered severely obese, i.e. having a BMI between 35 and 40 and at risk of obesity-related disease. The surgery usually involves shrinking the size of the stomach, meaning the amount of food a person can eat is limited. Gastric banding, which limits the capacity of the stomach using an inflatable band and causes an individual to feel full after only a small amount of food, is probably the most well-known type of weight loss surgery.

INDEX

Additional Resources

Other Issues titles

If you are interested in researching further some of the issues raised in *Staying Fit*, you may like to read the following titles in the **Issues** series:

⇨ Vol. 145 *Smoking Trends* (ISBN 978 1 86168 411 0)

⇨ Vol. 143 *Problem Drinking* (ISBN 978 1 86168 409 7)

⇨ Vol. 141 *Mental Health* (ISBN 978 1 86168 407 3)

⇨ Vol. 140 *Vegetarian and Vegan Diets* (ISBN 978 1 86168 406 6)

⇨ Vol. 127 *Eating Disorders* (ISBN 978 1 86168 366 3)

⇨ Vol. 125 *Understanding Depression* (ISBN 978 1 86168 364 9)

⇨ Vol. 123 *Young People and Health* (ISBN 978 1 86168 362 5)

⇨ Vol. 118 *Focus on Sport* (ISBN 978 1 86168 351 9)

⇨ Vol. 117 *Self-Esteem and Body Image* (ISBN 978 1 86168 350 2)

⇨ Vol. 100 *Stress and Anxiety* (ISBN 978 1 86168 314 4)

⇨ Vol. 88 *Food and Nutrition* (ISBN 978 1 86168 289 5)

⇨ Vol. 81 *Alternative Therapies* (ISBN 978 1 86168 276 5)

For more information about these titles, visit our website at www.independence.co.uk/publicationslist

Useful organisations

You may find the websites of the following organisations useful for further research:

⇨ **British Heart Foundation:** www.bhf.org.uk

⇨ **Bupa:** www.bupa.co.uk

⇨ **Cancer Research UK:** www.cancerresearch.org

⇨ **Channel 4:** www.channel4.com

⇨ **Department of Health:** www.dh.gov.uk

⇨ **Directgov:** www.direct.gov.uk

⇨ **Disordered Eating:** www.disordered-eating.co.uk

⇨ **Economic and Social Research Council:** www.esrcsocietytoday.ac.uk

⇨ **Foresight:** www.foresight.gov.uk

⇨ **NetDoctor:** www.netdoctor.co.uk

⇨ **Nuffield Proactive Health:** www.nuffieldproactivehealth.com

⇨ **The NHS:** www.ic.nhs.uk

⇨ **University of Bristol:** www.bristol.ac.uk

⇨ **University of Leeds:** www.leeds.ac.uk

⇨ **World Heart Federation:** www.world-heart-federation.org

ACKNOWLEDGEMENTS

The publisher is grateful for permission to reproduce the following material.

While every care has been taken to trace and acknowledge copyright, the publisher tenders its apology for any accidental infringement or where copyright has proved untraceable. The publisher would be pleased to come to a suitable arrangement in any such case with the rightful owner.

Chapter One: Unfit Britain

Obesity, © NetDoctor, *The politics of obesity*, © politics.co.uk, *Statistics on obesity, physical activity and diet*, © Crown copyright is reproduced with the permission of Her Majesty's Stationery Office, *Obesity worldwide*, © World Heart Federation, *Fat attack*, © Channel 4, *Genetic risk of obesity*, © Guardian Newspapers Ltd, *Sleepwalking towards obesity*, © Crown copyright is reproduced with the permission of Her Majesty's Stationery Office, *Busy lifestyles cause a death every 15 minutes*, © British Heart Foundation, *Fitness and ageing*, © Adfero, *Childhood obesity: a class and a classroom issue*, © Economic and Social Research Council, *Eleven-year-olds not taking enough exercise*, © University of Bristol, *Persecuting chubby kids*, © Guardian Newspapers Ltd.

Chapter Two: Fitness Solutions

The fitness strategy, © Crown copyright is reproduced with the permission of Her Majesty's Stationery Office, *Tackling obesities: future choices*, © Crown copyright is reproduced with the permission of Her Majesty's Stationery Office, *Surgery and drugs not enough to combat obesity*, © University of Bristol, *Obesity discrimination*, © Personnel Today, *Obesity in the workplace*, © Nuffield Proactive Health, *Obesity crisis: get paid to lose weight*, © Telegraph Group Ltd, *Make all staff exercise for an hour, says health adviser*, © 2008 Associated Newspapers Ltd, *Fitness barriers broken in workplace exercise trial*, © University of Leeds, *Avoiding childhood obesity*, © Bupa, *Treat childhood obesity as act of neglect, say doctors*, © Guardian Newspapers Ltd, *The answer to childhood obesity*, © University of Bristol, *Exercise 'does not make obese children slim'*, © Telegraph Group Ltd, *Physical activity*, © Bupa, *Reasons not to exercise*, © NetDoctor, *The fitness myths*, © Guardian Newspapers Ltd, *Keep-fit boom fails to stem obesity*, © This is London, *Study tips the scales in favour of exercise*, © University of Leeds, *Boost mental health*, © TheSite, *Obesity risk for 'moderately active' Britons*, © Adfero Ltd, *Exercise on par with drugs for aiding depression*, © Reuters, *Compulsive exercise*, © Disordered Eating.

Photographs

Stock Xchng: pages 3 (Laura Nubuck); 8 (Geo Cristian); 14, 39 (Steve Woods); 19 (Phil Edon, Richard Sweet, Manu M, Carlos Gustavo Curado); 31 (Xavi Sanchez).
Wikimedia Commons: page 9 (FatM1ke).

Illustrations

Pages 1, 16, 27, 33: Simon Kneebone; pages 4, 17, 28, 35: Angelo Madrid; pages 11, 20, 30, 38: Don Hatcher; pages 13, 22: Bev Aisbett.

Research and additional editorial by Claire Owen, on behalf of Independence Educational Publishers.

And with thanks to the team: Mary Chapman, Sandra Dennis, Claire Owen and Jan Sunderland.

Lisa Firth
Cambridge
September, 2008